D. Both · K. Frischknecht
Breastfeeding: An Illustrated Guide to Diagnosis and Treatment

Denise Both MSc, IBCLC has extensive experience as a breastfeeding and lactation consultant, including with the La Leche League. Denise has also published in various journals and is editor of the *European Journal for Breastfeeding and Lactation*. She teaches research interpretation and statistics in continuing education programs for the IBCLC, and is currently studying human medicine at the University of Ulm, Germany.

Kerri Frischknecht RN, RM, IBCLC, has more than 25 years' clinical experience in neonatal intensive care nursing in Australia and Switzerland, and established the first Swiss lactation program in a children's hospital. Kerri is author of numerous articles on breastfeeding, and co-authored a booklet for mothers with pre-term and sick newborns. She is an international conference speaker, is widely involved in breastfeeding and lactation education and has, since 2006, been the Swiss delegate for European Donor Milk Banks.

Denise Both · Kerri Frischknecht

Breastfeeding

An Illustrated Guide to Diagnosis and Treatment

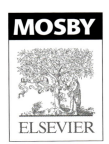

Sydney   Edinburgh   London   New York   Philadelphia   St Louis   Toronto

Mosby is an imprint of Elsevier

Elsevier Australia
(a division of Reed International Books Australia Pty Ltd)
30–52 Smidmore Street, Marrickville, NSW 2204
ACN 001 002 357

German edition © Urban & Fisher 2007
English translation © Elsevier Australia 2008

> This edition of Stillen kompakt. Atlas zur Diagnostik und Therapie in der Stillberatung by Denise Both & Kerri Frischknecht is published by arrangement with Elsevier GmbH, Urban & Fischer.
>
> The translation into English was undertaken by Elsevier Australia.
>
> German edition ISBN: 978 3 437 27460 2

This publication is copyright. Except as expressly provided in the Copyright Act 1968 and the Copyright Amendment (Digital Agenda) Act 2000, no part of this publication may be reproduced, stored in any retrieval system or transmitted by any means (including electronic, mechanical, microcopying, photocopying, recording or otherwise) without prior written permission from the publisher.

Every attempt has been made to trace and acknowledge copyright, but in some cases this may not have been possible. The publisher apologises for any accidental infringement and would welcome any information to redress the situation.

This publication has been carefully reviewed and checked to ensure that the content is as accurate and current as possible at time of publication. We would recommend, however, that the reader verify any procedures, treatments, drug dosages or legal content described in this book. Neither the author, the contributors, nor the publisher assume any liability for injury and/or damage to persons or property arising from any error in or omission from this publication.

National Library of Australia Cataloguing-in-Publication Data

Both, Denise.

Stillen kompakt. English

Breastfeeding : an illustrated guide to diagnosis and
treatment / authors, Denise Both ; Kerri Frischknecht.

Marrickville, N.S.W. : Elsevier Australia, 2008.

ISBN: 978 0 7295 3888 6 (hbk.).

Translated from German.

Breastfeeding–Handbooks, manuals, etc.
Breastfeeding–Complications.

Frischknecht, Kerri.

613.269

Publishing Editor: Debbie Lee
Publishing Services Manager: Helena Klijn
Translated by Web-Translations Ltd
Australian Editor: Deborah McRitchie
Typeset by DiZign
Printed by 1010 Printing International Ltd

    denotes reference.

    denotes cross reference to another figure in the publication.

Foreword

A mother who exclusively breastfeeds her baby uses approximately 25% of her daily energy expenditure for the production of breastmilk. This large commitment of energy to breastfeeding (greater than the proportion of energy used by the brain) shows, that during evolution, breastfeeding became vitally important to human survival. This conclusion is clearly supported today by research showing that, compared with formula fed babies, the mortality rate for breastfed babies is much lower in both developing and developed countries. This finding is not surprising because it is now known that breastmilk not only provides nourishment that is tailored to the developmental needs of the baby but also has an equally, if not more important role of providing innate immunological protection against pathogenic microorganisms. Furthermore, breastfeeding itself brings the mother and baby into a close contact that has been found to have subtle influences on positive physiological responses in both the mother and her baby.

For reasons that are hard to explain, in the past, affluent European women chose to have their babies wet-nursed. Indeed, Carl Linnaeus not only developed a new way of classifying plants and animals in the middle of the 18th century but also was against the popular practice of wet nursing babies. Therefore, he chose the term mammal, in preference to several alternatives, because he wanted to emphasise that these animals produced milk to feed their *own* young. At about the same time, in an essay to the governors of the Foundling Hospital in London, William Cadogan (1748) marvelled that poor women had no difficulty in breastfeeding their babies. He stated:

> *"The mother who has only a few rags to cover her baby loosely, and little more than her own breast to feed it, sees it healthy and strong, and very soon able to shift for itself,......"*

During the early 20th century as the level of affluence of the general population increased there was a greater demand for the limited number of wet nurses. At about this time, the mortality rate in Foundling hospitals was 50%–90% for babies fed cow's milk and it was found that pasteurisation of cow's milk greatly improved infant survival. Thus, increasing numbers of 'affluent' mothers resorted to using the 'pocket wet nurse' (bottle feeding) to nourish their babies with crudely modified cow's milk (infant 'formula'). Bottle feeding gained in popularity and became the accepted norm for infant feeding by the middle of the 20th century. Since 1972 in Australia and other developed countries, the proportion of mothers choosing to breastfeed their babies has gradually increased and, in contrast to Linnaeus and Cadogan's time, it is now the more affluent mothers who choose to breastfeed and the less affluent choose to feed infant formula. However, the breastfeeding environment for mothers today is substantially different to that of the poor women that Cadogan described.

As with other mammals, the newborn baby has the inherent skill to enable it to recognise the areola/nipple area and to suckle the breast. However, the new mother must acquire the skills required to correctly position and attach her baby to her breast. For the mother, breastfeeding skills are learned from previous experience as girls watching either their own mother or relatives breastfeed. Due to the small proportion of women choosing to breastfeed in the middle of the 20th century and the current social pressures against casual breastfeeding in public, current mothers have been deprived of the opportunity to subtly learn how to breastfeed their babies. Even successfully breastfeeding a baby does not provide a mother with a range of experiences that may be needed to successfully breastfeed her next child. Therefore, it has become the daunting task of today's health professionals, particularly midwives and lactation consultants, to teach in a few hours the skills women would have unconsciously acquired from observation and caring responsibilities associated with growing up in traditional societies.

Kerri Frischknecht and Denise Both have provided a clearly illustrated, easy to read book that provides an introduction to the latest research in breastfeeding and its application to resolving a broad range of practical problems that women encounter when breastfeeding their babies. The careful choice of pictorial material to illustrate the text has been made possible by the authors' wide experience in the field and ensures that the book will be a valuable resource for both health professional and mothers.

Professor Peter Hartmann
The University of Western Australia

Contents

1 Basic information about breastfeeding 1

1.1. The breast before, during and after pregnancy and lactation 2
1.1.1 Anatomy and physiology of the breast 2
1.1.2 Adolescence 3
1.1.3 Young, non-pregnant woman 3
1.1.4 Pregnant 3
1.1.5 Before birth 4
1.1.6 Lactation 4
1.1.7 Menopause 6

1.2 Normal course of breastfeeding 7
1.2.1 Breastfeeding initiation 7
1.2.2 Sequence of a breastfeed 9
1.2.3 Let-down reflex (milk ejection reflex) 12
1.2.4 Infant behavioural cues 13
1.2.5 Breastfeeding positions 14

1.3 Breastfeeding multiple infants 17

1.4 The older breastfed child 18

1.5 Tandem breastfeeding 19

1.6 Appearance of breast milk 19
1.6.1 Colostrum 19
1.6.2 Transitional milk 20
1.6.3 Mature breast milk 20
1.6.4 Blood in breast milk 20

1.7 Elimination, stool and urine output in the newborn 21
1.7.1 Meconium 21
1.7.2 Transitional stools 21
1.7.3 Breast milk stools 21
1.7.4 Stools from formula fed infants 22
1.7.5 Bloody stools 23
1.7.6 Urine 23

2 Breastfeeding problems and their causes 25

2.1 Atypical breast shapes 26
2.1.1 Asymmetric breasts 26
2.1.2 Inadequate mammary gland tissue 26
2.1.2 Accessory mammary gland tissue 27
2.1.4 Following breast surgery 28

2.2. Problematic nipple forms 30
2.2.1 Flat nipples 30
2.2.2 Retracted/inverted nipples 31
2.2.3 Small nipples 33
2.2.4 Large nipples 33
2.2.5 Bifurcated or double nipples 33

2.3 Pathological changes of the breast 34
2.3.1 Mammary gland swelling (initial engorgement) 34
2.3.2 Local engorgement (plugged ducts) 34
2.3.3 Mastitis 35
2.3.4 Abscess 35
2.3.5 Breast cancer 36
2.3.6 Nipple cancer (Paget's disease of the nipple) . 36

2.4 Pain and injury of the nipple 37
2.4.1 Sore nipples 37
2.4.2 Nipple fissures 37
2.4.3 *Candida*/thrush 38
2.4.4 Psoriasis 38
2.4.5 Allergic reactions 39
2.4.6 Virus infections – Herpes 39
2.4.7 Raynaud's phenomenon/vasospasm 40
2.4.8 Milk bleb/milk blisters 40
2.4.9 Bacterial infections 40

2.5 Lifestyle 41
2.5.1 Tattoos 41
2.5.2 Piercing 41

2.6	**Infants with special needs**	42	3.2.2 Breast shells (B) for protection	68
2.6.1	Prematurity	42	3.2.3 Niplette	68
2.6.2	Respiratory problems	49	3.2.4 Nipple shields	68

2.6 Infants with special needs 42
2.6.1 Prematurity 42
2.6.2 Respiratory problems 49
2.6.3 Reflux 50
2.6.4 Down syndrome 50
2.6.5 Neurological impairment 51
2.6.6 Cephalhaematoma (caput succedaneum) ... 51
2.6.7 Failure to thrive 52
2.6.8 Cleft lip, cleft of the upper alveolar ridge (gum) and palate 52
2.6.9 Pierre Robin sequence 54
2.6.10 Choanal atresia and stenosis 55
2.6.11 Ankyloglossia 56
2.6.12 Oral candidiasis 57
2.6.13 Neonatal icterus (jaundice) 57
2.6.14 Cardiac defects 58
2.6.15 Chylothorax 58
2.6.16 Haemangioma 58

3 Breastfeeding aids and alternative feeding methods 59

3.1 Aids for expressing human breast milk .. 60
3.1.1 Breast pumps 60
3.1.2 Breast massage 64
3.1.3 Equipment for transport and storage ... 65

3.2 Devices for nipples 67
3.2.1 Breast shells (A) for inverted nipples 67
3.2.2 Breast shells (B) for protection ... 68
3.2.3 Niplette 68
3.2.4 Nipple shields 68

3.3. Alternative feeding methods for the infant 70
3.3.1 Cup feeding 70
3.3.2 Soft feeder 71
3.3.3 Spoon 72
3.3.4 Pipette 72
3.3.5 Supplementary nursing system 72
3.3.6 Finger feeding 74
3.3.7 Haberman Feeder (Special Needs Feeder) 75
3.3.8 Bottle feeding 76
3.3.9 Pacifiers 76

3.4 Personal hygiene and clothing 76
3.4.1 Nursing pads 76
3.4.2 Temperature packs 77
3.4.3 Ointments 77
3.4.4 Nursing bra 78

Appendix 79
Glossary 80
References 83
Addresses 86
Websites 87
Index 88

Photograph and diagram references

The respective photograph and diagram reference sources are situated beneath each picture plate at the end of the figure legend in square brackets.

F212: Cooper, A. P.: Anatomy of the breast. London: Longman, Orme, Green, Brown and Longmans, 1840.

E281: Egli, F.: Frischknecht, K; Geborgenheit Liebe und Muttermilch. Ein Ratgeber für Eltern von Frühgeborenen und kranken Neugeborenen, rund ums Stillen, Anpumpen und Muttermilch. Sarnen: Balance Verlag 2002 & 2004 (Security, Love and Mother's Milk. A guide for parents of premature and sick newborn infants: comprehensive aspects regarding breastfeeding and milk expression. Sarnen: Balance Publishers, 2002, 2004).

M307: Kerri Frischknecht, RN, RM, Breastfeeding and Lactation Consultant IBCLC, Herisau, Switzerland.

M308: Franziska Egli, Breastfeeding and Lactation Consultant IBCLC, Stans, Switzerland.

0442: Mark Fallander.

0443: Alexander Kuehne, Switzerland.

0444: Erik Zubler, Switzerland.

0445: Christa Herzog, Breastfeeding and Lactation Consultant IBCLC, Lucerne, Switzerland.

T346: Professor Renzo Brun del Re, Switzerland.

T347: Dr. Peter Donski, Specialist FMH for plastic, reconstructive and aesthetic surgery.

0446: Dr. Helmut Egger, Freudenberg, Germany.

0447: Dr. Lisa Amir, Australia.

0448: Norbert Lutsch, Switzerland.

0449: Dr. Jacqueline Kent, Australia.

T348: Dr. Peter Waibel, St. Gallen, Switzerland.

0450: Martina Jungbluth.

T349: Ramsay, D.; Langton, D.; Jacobs, L.; Gollow, I.; Simmer, K.; 2004

T350: Dr. Dagmar Klima-Lange, Paediatric Surgeon, St. Gallen, Switzerland.

Figure 3: With courtesy from Ramsay, D.T.; Hartmann, R.L.; Hartmann P.E.; Kent, J.C.

Introduction

'Breastfeeding is the most natural thing in the world.'
'Breastfeeding is important.'
'Every woman can breastfeed if she wants to.'

Women, pregnant women in particular, are confronted with these statements time and again. These ideas are considered by many to be so universal that they regard breastfeeding counselling as a speciality amounting to no more than a footnote in the medical field. It is precisely these people who are amazed to find out that there is specialised education for breastfeeding and lactation consultants and thick textbooks dealing with the subject.

Breastfeeding is certainly the most natural thing in the world. After all, mammals would have died out long ago if this way of nourishing offspring could only be mastered with a university degree. In spite of everything, breastfeeding is something that needs to be learned, by the mother as well as the infant. This learning process begins long before the delivery of the first child – at least it should do. But unfortunately it has become rare for knowledge about the art of breastfeeding to be passed down from mothers and grandmothers or other female relatives to the next generation. Often, her own first baby is the first infant that a woman sees or holds in her arms. She must therefore feel her way slowly in order to find out what it means to be a mother and how breastfeeding works.

Breastfeeding is important. This statement is supported scientifically, and for good reason the World Health Organization (WHO) recommends for all children exclusive breastfeeding for the first six months, followed by the continuation of breastfeeding with simultaneous introduction of solid foods appropriate for the infant's age until at least their second birthday and then for as long as the mother and child want. The health of both mother and child benefits from breastfeeding in many ways. Breastfeeding makes it easier for the woman to become accustomed to her new role as a mother and to build a good relationship with her child. This doesn't mean that women who don't breastfeed cannot establish a good bond with their children, but the hormonal state of a breastfeeding mother makes some things easier.

Every woman can breastfeed if she wants to. It is true that, from a purely organic point of view, between 95% and 98% of all women are capable of breastfeeding their infants. But there are still 2%–5% who want to breastfeed just as much and still, even after the best information and the most support possible, cannot breastfeed completely or at all. For these women, the expectation that every woman can breastfeed if she wants to is deeply hurtful. There are also women who are capable of breastfeeding their infants, but the infants are not able to breastfeed for various reasons. Then there are women whose path to breastfeeding seems like a hurdle race and who must overcome many problems in order to breastfeed their children – and some women are obliged to give up the race. For all these women, competent, sensitive support is important directly after delivery, during the early days at home, and also when the breastfed child is older, as problems can arise at any point during breastfeeding.

This book shows the normal course of breastfeeding – how it should be and how it actually is in the majority of cases. It also points out which problems can arise and suggests ways of helping to solve these problems. This book is therefore aimed at all those who work with mothers and babies – and who, in doing so, have an important task to fulfil.

1
Basic information about breastfeeding

1.1. The breast before, during and after pregnancy and lactation 2

1.2 Normal course of breastfeeding 7

1.3 Breastfeeding multiple infants 17

1.4 The older breastfed child 18

1.5 Tandem breastfeeding......................... 19

1.6 Appearance of breast milk 19

1.7 Elimination, stool and urine output in the newborn .. 21

1.1 The breast before, during and after pregnancy and lactation

1.1.1 Anatomy and physiology of the breast

Historical depiction

For more than 160 years, illustrations of breast anatomy were based on the investigations of the anatomist and surgeon Sir Astley Cooper. (1)
In 1840, Cooper injected hot, diversely coloured wax in the milk ducts of women, who had died when they were lactating. The wax casts were then arranged symmetrically as shown. However this arrangement does not necessarily reflect the true anatomical position of the milk ducts and other structures within the breast.

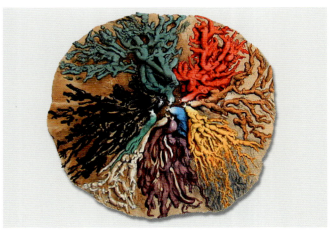

Fig. 1: Artistic representation of the anatomy of the breast according to Cooper with forced dilation of the milk ducts (2) [F212]

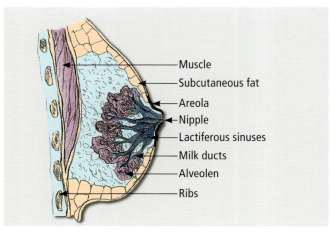

Fig. 2: Until recently, representations of breast anatomy corresponded largely to the illustrations of Cooper [E281]

Depiction of breast anatomy up until now

For decades, illustrations of the lactating breast shown in all textbooks followed the diagrams or descriptions made by Cooper. The strict symmetry of the breast structure is noteworthy. As a rule, 15 to 20 milk ducts were shown per breast, with the same number of ducts leading to the nipple. (1) The milk ducts extended to the so-called lactiferous sinus, which was considered to serve as a reservoir for the milk produced between the periods of breastfeeding. Cooper documented up to 22 milk ducts, but did not consider all of them to be functional. According to him, less than 12 patent ducts terminated at the nipple.

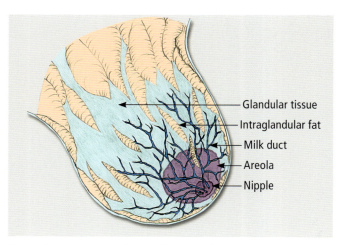

Fig. 3: More recent studies could not confirm the existence of lactiferous sinuses [E281]

Current depiction of breast anatomy

Curent research indicates that the distribution of glandular tissue is symmetrical between breasts, with medial aspects having less glandular tissue than lateral sections. Lactiferous sinuses are not apparent, all milk ducts branch within the areola radius, the first occuring 8.0 ± 5.5 mm from the base of the nipple. The function of the main milk ducts is transport not storage. Ducts have a tortuous path with diameters of 1.9 ± 0.6 mm in the left breast and 2.0 ± 0.7 mm in the right. The number of main ducts is 9.6 ± 2.9 and 9.2 ± 2.9 mm for left and right breasts respectively. Adipose tissue is distributed between lobes. (3)

1.1.2 Adolescence

The first stage of breast development, embryogenesis, begins before birth. From about 18 to 19 weeks' gestation, an epithelial mammary bud is present. This bud grows in the mammary fat pad and the milk ducts have blind endings. Following birth, these small ducts grow as the child grows. The pubertal development of the breast starts some time before menarche and, alongside the extension of the milk ducts, also results in visible external growth of the breast.

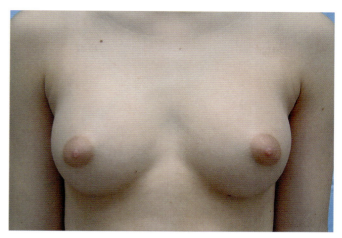

Fig. 4: Typical appearance of the breast of a 14-year-old teenager one year after menarche [M307]

1.1.3 Young, non-pregnant woman

From pre-puberty the milk ducts differentiate further under the influence of oestrogen and growth hormones. Furthermore, glandular end-buds (acini) develop, within which the alveoli will form during subsequent development. Following puberty, each menstrual cycle will affect the breast. Progesterone in particular may have a significant influence on the development of alveoli and lobules. (📖 4)

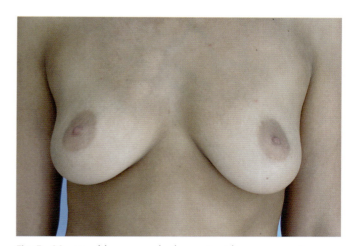

Fig. 5: 20-year-old woman who has not yet been pregnant [M307]

1.1.4 Pregnant

During pregnancy, placental and luteal hormones stimulate proliferation and branching of the milk ducts and thus further development of the lobes. Placental lactogen, prolactin and chorionic gonadotrophin are also conducive to increased growth. Lactogenesis I begins about halfway through pregnancy. From this time onwards, milk production is possible in principle, however this will still be suppressed by pregnancy hormones. (📖 5) Figures 6, 7 and 8 show the breast changes at different gestational stages in the same woman.

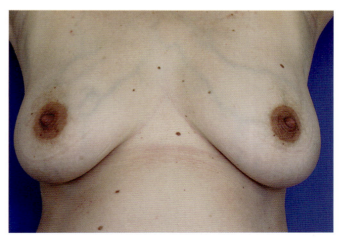

Fig. 6: 21st week of pregnancy: the pregnancy-induced changes in the breast are noticeable [M307]

1.1 The breast before, during and after pregnancy and lactation

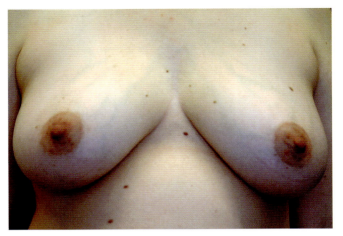

Fig. 7: 38th week of pregnancy: the breast has increased in size and weight [M307]

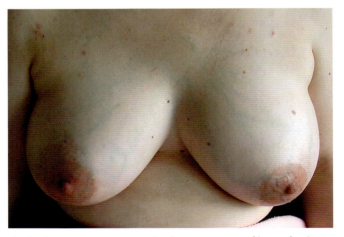

Fig. 8: Day 4 postpartum: optimal management of breastfeeding prevents problems during the initial coming-in of milk [M307]

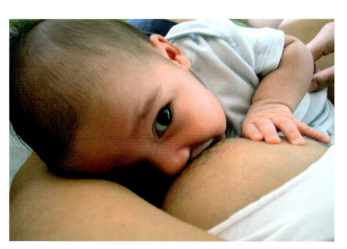

Fig. 9: Mother and child get to know each other increasingly better [O442]

1.1.5 Before birth

The glandular tissue has increasingly displaced the connective and fatty tissue, making the breast look heavier and fuller. However, the proportion of fat remains the same. The areola has increased in size, and the nipples and areola are more strongly pigmented. The Montgomery glands are more prominent and venous patterns are clearly visible. Many mothers have already been secreting colostrum for some time. Delivery of the placenta is a signal for milk production to start. (⌇ 6) Figs. 6, 7 and 8 show the same woman.

1.1.6 Lactation

Engorgement (initial coming-in of milk lactogenesis II)

From about the 2nd to 5th day postpartum, a swelling of the breasts occurs, which indicates the onset of copious milk secretion. It is important to know that the degree of tissue swelling is not correlated with milk quantity and that frequent and unrestricted breastfeeding is important for the initial coming-in of the milk to proceed without complications. If breastfeeding occurs too infrequently, the initial physiological coming-in of milk can develop into a pathological engorgement of the mammary glands. (☞ Fig. 87, 88)

Well established nursing relationship

It takes about six weeks before the mother and child get used to each other and a good nursing relationship is established. Especially in the very first weeks, it is important for the mother and child to spend time together to bond and to learn to breastfeed in a relaxed and unhurried atmosphere. Stressful situations, for example the cluster feeding typical of young infants (frequent, short episodes of breastfeeding that are only interrupted by short phases of sleep and can last for several hours), will soon belong to the past, and often a routine is established.

The feeling of tightness that often occurs at the commencement of lactation usually subsides after a few weeks. The breasts will become softer and, in many women, will also become somewhat smaller again. When the child is thriving, this does not indicate a decrease in milk production, but rather that the nursing relationship has become well established. At this point the risk of sore nipples and other breastfeeding problems decreases, but the mother should continue to pay attention to good attachment and to a correct sucking pattern by her child.

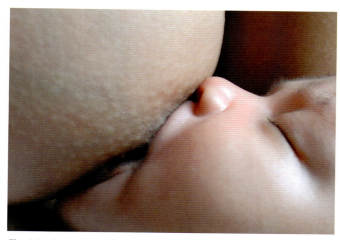

Fig. 10: Correct attachment and sucking are the key to a successful breastfeeding relationship [O442]

Weaning

Weaning commences as soon as the infant is no longer exclusively breastfed. In the ideal case, a child will indicate its readiness for supplementary food about halfway through the first year of life. As soon as the infant signals that they want more than breast milk, solid food is offered slowly and in gradually increasing quantities. At the same time, the child should continue to be breastfed at least until their second birthday. (☞ 7) In principal, lactation could be maintained indefinitely as long as the breasts are stimulated.

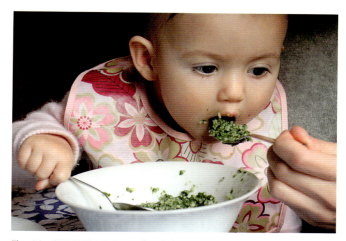

Fig. 11: SUPPLEMENTARY food should initially be understood literally: it supplements breast milk [O443]

If the breasts are no longer regularly stimulated, involution begins. In this phase of lactation, the composition of the milk changes (e.g. the sodium content increases). The resulting change in the taste of the milk can even make weaning easier. Not only does the child profit from a long period of breastfeeding, but longer periods of breastfeeding have a long-term positive influence on maternal bone density (☞ 8–10) and is protective against certain forms of cancer. (☞ 11)

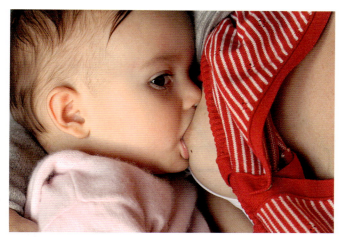

Fig. 12: Weaning starts as soon as a child receives solid food or milk formula [O443]

1.1 The breast before, during and after pregnancy and lactation

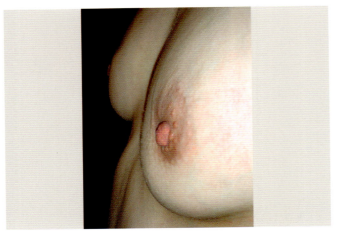

Fig. 13: Many women are shocked by the appearance of their breasts immediately after weaning [M308]

In the initial period following weaning, the breasts may seem smaller and flabbier. After a few menstrual cycles, the breasts gradually regain their firmness. In rare cases, some mothers can have a transient loss of fat that used to be present in their breasts before pregnancy. This fat gradually develops again with time, although only if the woman has not lost a lot of weight permanently.

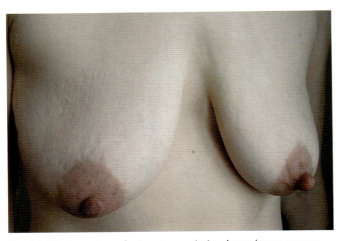

Fig. 14: The breast needs time to regain its shape (same woman as in Fig. 65) [M307]

In the long term, breastfeeding does not have any influence on the form or appearance of the breasts. Some time after weaning, it is no longer possible to tell whether a woman has ever breastfed, only whether she was pregnant. The lasting changes in the breasts are not associated with breastfeeding but with pregnancy. Women with weak connective tissue will notice more changes than women with very firm connective tissue.

1.1.7 Menopause

During the menopause, the breasts also change. The cycle-dependent stimulation of the breasts is completed, the glandular tissue reduces and the percentage of fat increases. The breasts increasingly lose firmness and become more flaccid. Since the breast tissue is less dense after menopause than in a young women, breast investigations using imaging procedures such as mammography are simpler.

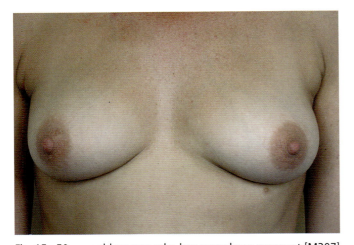

Fig. 15: 50-year-old woman who has never been pregnant [M307]

Comparison of Figures 15 and 16 shows that, during menopause, there are hardly any differences between the breasts of women of the same age, comparable body weight, percentage of fatty tissue and connective tissue of similar quality, regardless of whether or not they have breastfed.

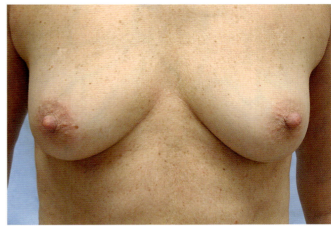

Fig. 16: 50-year-old multiparous woman, gravida 5/para 3, three children breastfed for a total of three years [M307]

The percentage of fatty tissue and the quality of the connective tissue as well as the general body stature and genetic disposition also determine the appearance of the breasts after menopause.

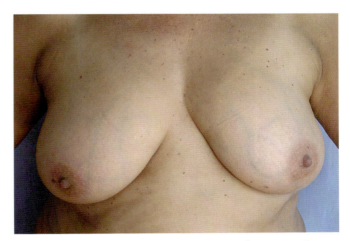

Fig. 17: 60-year-old multiparous woman, gravida 4/para 4, four children breastfed for a total of a little over six years [M307]

1.2 Normal course of breastfeeding

1.2.1 Breastfeeding initiation

During pregnancy, the breast is prepared for breastfeeding. However, milk production continues to be largely suppressed until delivery. This suppression is predominantly due to high levels of progesterone (determined by the placenta), to the occupation of prolactin receptors by human placental lactogen (HPL) as well as to the effect of prolactin-inhibiting factors (PIF). Following delivery of the placenta, there is an abrupt decrease in the levels of oestrogen, progesterone, HPL and PIF. The prolactin level rises markedly and prolactin binds to the receptors that are no longer blocked by HPL. This is the starting signal for lactogenesis II. (6)

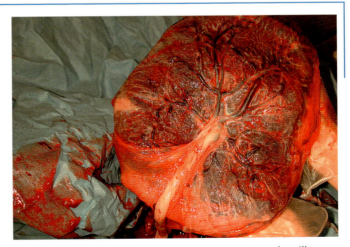

Fig. 18: Remnants of placenta in the uterus can impede milk production [O443]

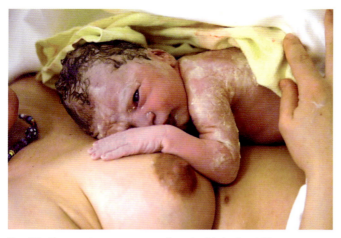

Fig. 19: The precious moments after the birth should be as undisturbed as possible [O444]

Following birth, the newborn should have the opportunity to lie undisturbed skin-to-skin with the mother and enter into the world in its own time. Fully awake, it finds its way to the breast and independently takes the nipple into its mouth. This first interaction between mother and newborn should be as undisturbed as possible. The physical contact between the mother and infant stimulates the mother to release prolactin and oxytocin, supports thermoregulation and metabolism in the infant and, furthermore, forms the foundation for a good breastfeeding relationship.

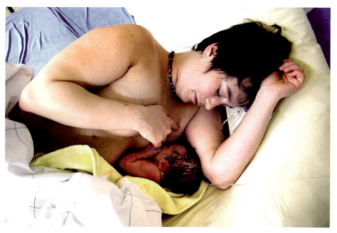

Fig. 20: Frequent, unrestricted and early nursing, already in delivery room, prevents breastfeeding problems [O444]

Early and frequent nursing without time limitations inhibits the secretion of PIF and stimulates the mother to release prolactin. This ensures that a sufficient number of prolactin receptors is occupied and optimal milk production occurs. In these first days, milk production is subject to endocrine regulation and is independent of the breast being emptied. The continuation of milk production, lactogenesis III, is regulated through autocrine mechanisms, that is the stimulation and emptying of the breast. (📖 12)

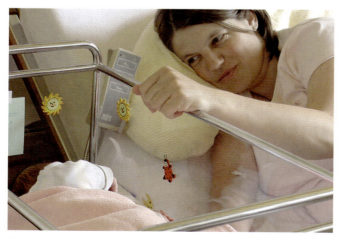

Fig. 21: Rooming-in offers many advantages for mother and newborn [M307]

Rooming-in

For many years it was common practice to separate mother and infant after birth. The intention was that the mother should rest and the newborn should be protected from harmful germs. It was not recognised for a long time that the separation of mother and infant had precisely the opposite effect. The separation of mother and infant leaves the newborn open to colonisation by pathogenic organisms and does not assist the mother's recovery. (📖 13, 14)

Rooming-in enables breastfeeding to take place on demand at any time, including at night. Unrestricted and frequent nursing promotes milk production and prevents problems during the initial coming-in of the milk (☞ 1.1.6). 24-hour rooming-in is the best prophylaxis against breastfeeding problems, it promotes frequent breastfeeding, reduces the need for supplementary feeds, has a positive effect on the total duration of breastfeeding and supports bonding. (📖 13, 15)

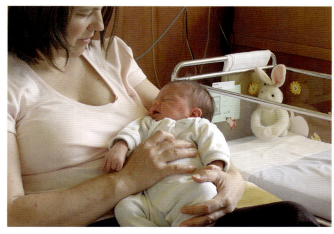

Fig. 22: Undisturbed communication between mother and child gives the mother more confidence [M307]

If the mother reacts promptly to early signs of hunger in the newborn (☞ 1.2.2), the infant cries less, expends less energy and loses less weight. Mothers who stay with their newborns sleep more peacefully and thus are more rested. Mother and newborn get to know each other better and, above all, first-time mothers gain confidence in handling their child. This eases the adjustment to daily life at home.

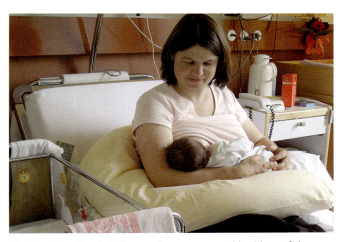

Fig. 23: Rooming-in helps mothers to rest and builds confidence in their mothering abilities [M307]

1.2.2 Sequence of a breastfeed

For a long time, breastfeeding according to fixed schedules was promoted. This led to early weaning because of 'reduced milk supply'. After the recommendation for breastfeeding on demand (ad libitum) had become more or less accepted, the crying of the infant was often considered to be a signal for the next breastfeed. In many cases, it is not taken into consideration how very difficult it can be to put a fussy crying infant, to the breast.

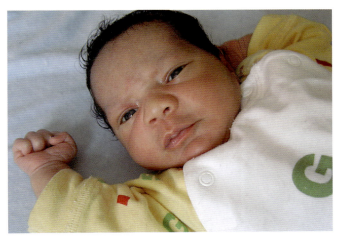

Fig. 24: The active alert state is the optimal time for a breastfeed to take place or commence [M307]

1.2 Normal course of breastfeeding

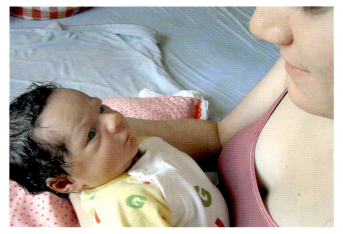

Fig. 25: During breastfeeding there is a special interaction between mother and infant [M307]

An optimal starting point for a breastfeed is provided by behavioural cues: sucking movements, sucking noises, licking of the lips, rapid eye movements, the head turning from side to side (searching movements), restlessness, movements of the arms and legs. After the first four weeks, the child putting its finger or hand into their mouth is no longer a reliable hunger cue. The infant is now beginning to explore themselves and their environment, and the mouth plays an important role here.

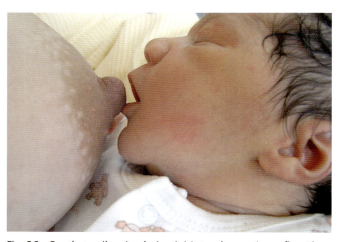

Fig. 26: Gentle tactile stimulation initiates the rooting reflex. The infant turns towards the nipple [M307]

Oral reactions/reflexes

The reflexes stimulated by contact, such as the rooting and sucking reflexes, cause the infant to seek nourishment. Protective oral reflexes, for example the gagging and coughing reflex enable safe drinking without aspiration. (📖 16) A healthy, full term neonate is able to coordinate sucking, swallowing and breathing and drink from the breast without difficulties. If this is not the case, the infant must be examined thoroughly.

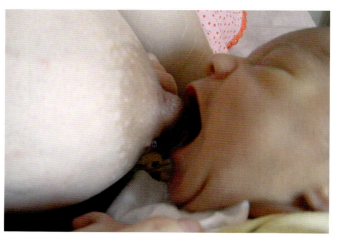

Fig. 27: The mouth is wide open to take in the breast, like a 'hungry bird' [M307]

After the child has turned to the nipple with its mouth and touched the nipple with the lower lip, the reflex to open the mouth is stimulated. The infant opens its mouth wide, as if yawning. If the mouth is not open wide enough, correct attachment is not possible. The consequences of poor attachment can be sore nipples and inadequate emptying of the breast and thus an insufficient stimulation of milk production.

Correct attachment/latch-on

The infant drinks in a rhythmic pattern with regular pauses. It should be possible to hear or see the swallowing. Towards the end of the breastfeed, the pauses become longer and the infant may possibly release the nipple. The mother notices that her breasts feel less heavy.

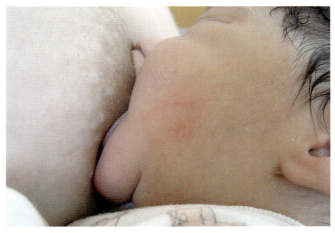

Fig. 28: Optimal attachment: the lips are rolled outwards, there is hardly any or no space between nose and breast [M307]

Incorrect attachment

In comparison to an infant who is well attached with a good latch-on technique, a poorly attached child may put on insufficient weight and the mother may suffer from sore or cracked, abraded nipples. On observation, the infant does not open their mouth wide enough, or only sucks the tip of the nipple rather than having a good part of the areola in their mouth. These infants often require frequent feeds and are very restless.

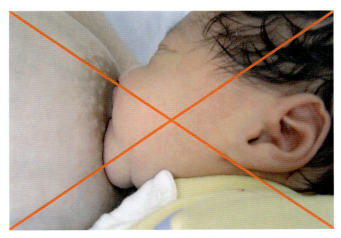

Fig. 29: INCORRECT attachment and sucking often lead to problems with breastfeeding [M307]

Completion of the breastfeed

No mandatory time period can be given for the duration of a breastfeed. Ideally, the breastfeed will last until the infant themself ends it. Younger infants usually feed longer than older babies. Towards the end of the breastfeed, the infant will suck and swallow less and less frequently. The baby has a more relaxed muscle tone, the hands are looser and the limbs become heavy. Finally, the infant lets go of the breast and will often fall asleep.

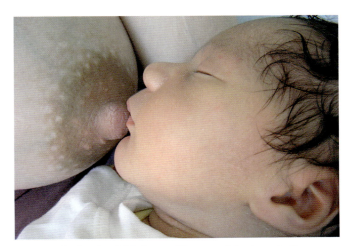

Fig. 30: Ideally, the child themself lets go of the breast after feeding [M307]

1.2 Normal course of breastfeeding

In the first weeks, the infant will feed, on average, approximately eight to twelve times in 24 hours. A breastfeed usually lasts until the child ends it. Whether one or both breasts are offered in a breastfeeding session always depends on the individual situation. In the first weeks it is usually advisable to offer both breasts, although it is not always necessary to do so in all circumstances . Each mother–child dyad must find its own way. The breastfeeding behaviour of the child can change at any time.

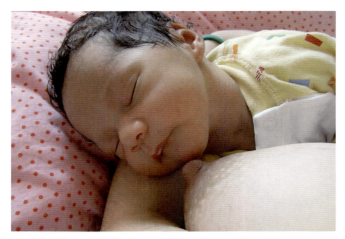

Fig. 31: After breastfeeding, the infant is relaxed or falls asleep [M307]

1.2.3 Let-down reflex (milk ejection reflex)

As soon as an infant sucks at the breast, nerve impulses are sent to the posterior lobe of the pituitary gland, resulting in oxytocin release. Due to contraction of the myoepithelial cells surrounding the alveoli, the milk is squeezed into the milk ducts so that it is available to the infant. The diameter of the milk ducts increases during the milk ejection reflex and remains dilated for up to two minutes. (👉 17)

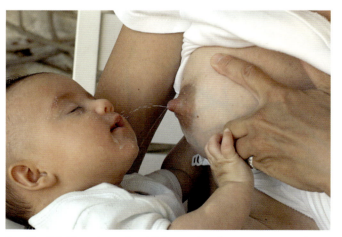

Fig. 32: Thinking about the child or seeing them can initiate the milk ejection reflex [O443]

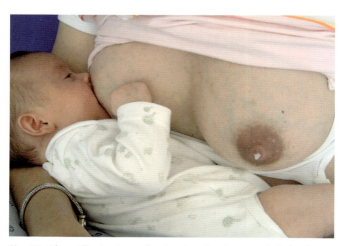

Fig. 33: The milk ejection reflex begins simultaneously in both breasts [O443]

Nearly 75% of all women experience more than one let-down reflex per breastfeed, the average being 2.5 milk ejection reflexes (range: 1–9). Before the start of the milk ejection reflex, the quantity of milk that flows is not large. Almost half of the infant's milk intake takes place during the first let-down reflex within a breastfeed. Some 33% of infants end the breastfeed after the first let-down reflex. Breastfeeding offers the best possibility for stimulating a milk ejection reflex. Mothers who express milk with a pump can require twice as much time for initiation of the reflex. If the milk is not emptied from the breast during the milk ejection reflex, it flows back into the milk ducts. (👉 17)

1.2.4 Infant behavioural cues

Infant states, also called the state of consciousness, affect the child's reactions at any given time. States are understood to mean behaviour and psychological characteristics that always recur according to a regular pattern (📖 18), including physical activity, movements of the eyes and face, patterns of breathing and reactions to stimulation. (📖 19)

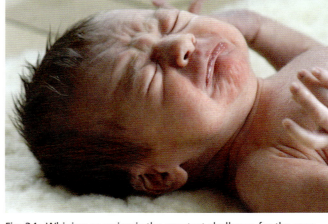

Fig. 34: Whining or crying is the greatest challenge for the care giver [O444]

The states of consciousness are usually divided into sleeping and awake states, which are further divided into subgroups. Certain states of consciousness enable the child to come to terms better with the stimuli to which it is exposed from its environment. (📖 16, 18, 19)

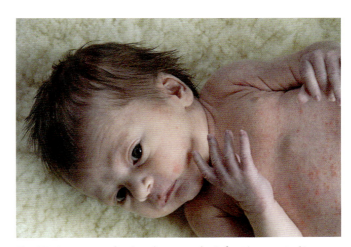

Fig. 35: In a state of quiet alertness, the infant is open to its environment [O444]

Feeding on demand according to the needs of the child, instead of according to a timetable, is the recommended way in which to nurse or feed an infant under normal circumstances. The mother or care giver decides, on the basis of various signals from the infant (☞ 1.2.2), when the infant will be fed. Crying is a very late sign of hunger.

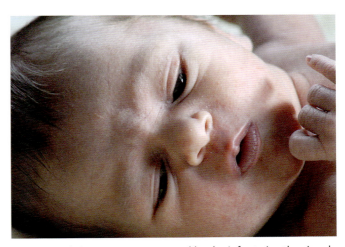

Fig. 36: Early hunger cues expressed by the infant give the signal for breastfeeding [O444]

1.2 Normal course of breastfeeding

1.2.5 Breastfeeding positions

A correct and comfortable position for breastfeeding is of prime importance for breastfeeding success. An optimal breastfeeding position is one that enables the women to feel comfortable and enables her child to relax while feeding. Incorrect attachment (☞ Fig. 29) can be the cause of tension, sore nipples (☞ 2.4), insufficient milk and, finally, premature weaning.

Many problems can be avoided if the child is attached correctly and the mother has found a breastfeeding position that is comfortable and suitable for herself and the child. In an infant that is attached properly in a correct breastfeeding position, the ear, shoulder and hip of the child form a straight line.

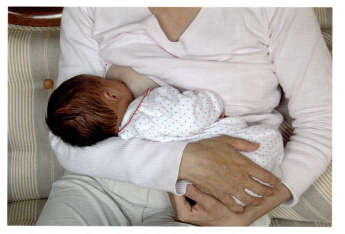

Fig. 37: The cradle position is the best known breastfeeding position [M307]

Cradle position

The cradle hold is the most traditional position. The woman sits upright, the head of the child rests on her forearm or in the bend of the elbow. The child lies on its side turned towards the mother and is drawn in close to her. The underneath arm of the child either lies under the woman's breast or around her waist. The shoulder and back of the women, as well as the arm holding the child, should be supported.

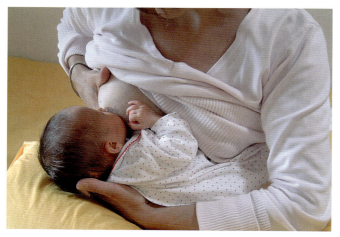

Fig. 38: Very suitable where there are attachment problems, engorgement and large breasts [M307]

Cross-cradle position

The woman sits upright and raises her child to breast height. If the right breast is offered, the right hand makes a U shape in order to support the breast. The left hand and left arm support the trunk, shoulders and head of the child. As soon as the infant opens its mouth, it can be drawn gently to the breast. This position is especially suitable for ill newborn and premature infants.

Football position

The woman sits upright. The body of the child lies sideways to her, so that the head and abdomen of the child are turned to the mother. The buttocks lie supported by a cushion near to the woman's elbow, the upper back lies parallel to the mother's supporting forearm. The back of the head is supported with the hand. The shoulders, back, forearm and possibly wrist of the woman should be supported. The position enables the best possible control over the head, neck and trunk of the child. This breastfeeding position is very suitable after caesarean section, during coming-in of milk and with engorgement, and well as for premature babies.

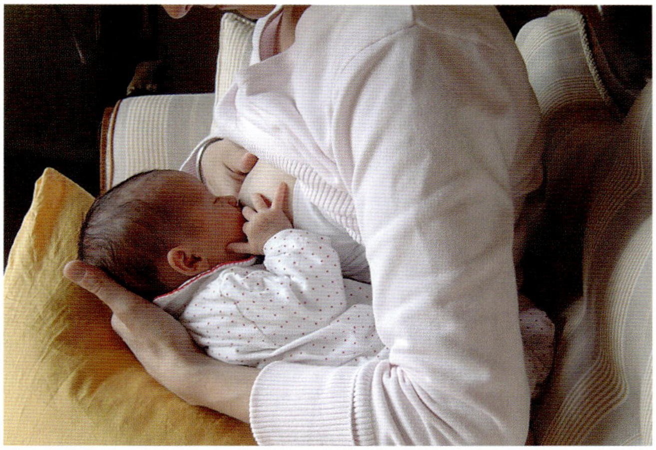

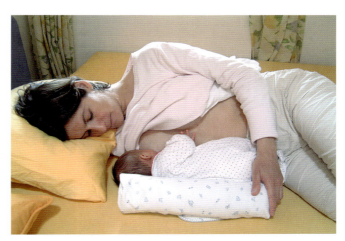

Fig. 39: The football position is especially suitable in the early days as well as for premature and sick infants [M307]

Side-lying position

Breastfeeding while lying down offers the woman the opportunity to rest while nursing, or even to sleep. Following caesarean section or episiotomy, the stitches are not put under strain in this position. Mother and child lie on their sides facing each other. The child's back is either supported by the upper arm of the mother or by a rolled-up towel. Cushions under the mother's head, behind her back and under the knee of the top leg can help her assume a comfortable position. The infant can feed from both breasts without the mother needing to turn.

Fig. 40: Breastfeeding while lying down offers the mother the opportunity to rest, or even to sleep while breastfeeding [M307]

Straddle position

The infant sits on the mother's knee, their face turned to the mother and legs to the right and left of her body. This position is beneficial when there is a strong milk ejection reflex, engorgement in the lower quadrants of the breast and possibly in the case of a child with cleft palate, since there is less flow of the milk into the nasal area in this position. Of course, a young infant must be very well supported.

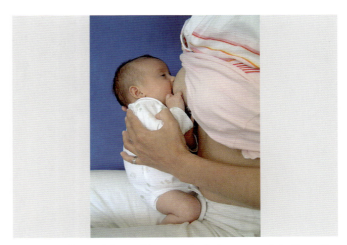

Fig. 41: In the upright position, gravity helps to regulate the milk flow [M307]

1.2 Normal course of breastfeeding

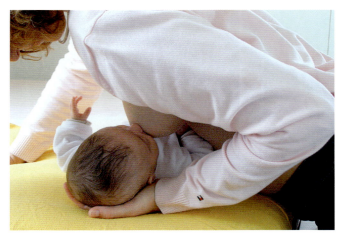

Fig. 42: Somewhat acrobatic, but effective [M307]

Leaning over position

The mother is on hands and knees in a leaning over position or standing leaning over, with the child lying on its back beneath her. The infant is raised to the appropriate height by a cushion or blanket. Ideally, the infant lies on a firm surface, for example on a bed. Depending on the location of the affected area, this position is suitable when there is engorgement. The infant should be attached in such a way that their chin points to the engorged site.

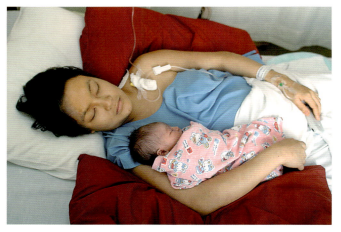

Fig. 43: Even after a caesarean section, the mother and child should not be separated [O442]

Breastfeeding after caesarean section

After a caesarean section, the coming-in of the milk is no different from that after a vaginal delivery. The signal for the initiation of milk secretion is given by the delivery of the placenta and not by labour. If lactogenesis II is delayed following a caesarean, this is almost always due to the fact that the mother and child were separated and that the child therefore did not have sufficient opportunity to feed early and frequently at the breast. If the infant is nursed unrestrictedly, as a rule breastfeeding proceeds no differently than after a vaginal delivery.

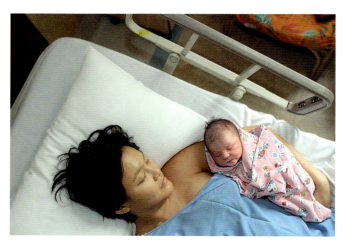

Fig. 44: After a caesarean section, breastfeeding while lying on the back or side is often recommended to relieve pain [O442]

If the caesarean was conducted under epidural anaesthesia, the mother can nurse the child as soon as the surgical wound has been closed. She should be supported in this by the nursing personnel or her partner. After general anaesthesia, breastfeeding can begin as soon as the mother is awake and able to hold her newborn by herself. (📖 20)

After a caesarean section, breastfeeding while lying on the back or side is usually recommended at first. In this way, the mother can breastfeed fairly comfortably and with less pain despite the abdominal incision. A bed with side bars and pillows to support the mother is very helpful in these cases.

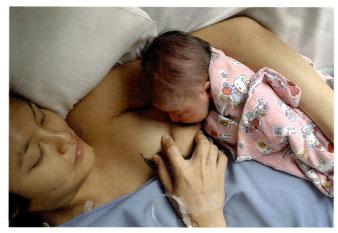

Fig. 45: A sufficiently wide bed perhaps with side rails is optimal for breastfeeding lying on the back [O442]

1.3 Breastfeeding multiple infants

Breastfeeding more than one infant is possible and most mothers are biologically capable of producing enough milk for at least two children. However, multiple pregnancies more often lead to premature birth and a higher rate of caesarean section, which can hinder the initiation of breastfeeding in particular. Women expecting more than one child therefore need further support and advice in addition to the basic information about breastfeeding. Ideally, the expectant mother is placed under the care of a breastfeeding and lactation consultant prior to delivery.

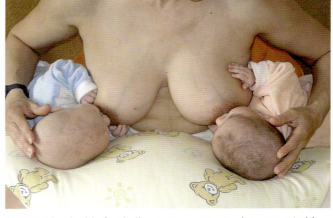

Fig. 46: The double football or twin position is also very suitable after a caesarean section [M307]

If the children are healthy and stable, they should, like all other newborn babies, be nursed as soon as possible after the delivery and breastfed frequently and without restrictions. If relocation of the children is necessary, or if they are unable to adequately nurse from the breast, milk expression should be started as soon as possible (☞ 2.6.1) in order to initiate milk production and stimulate an ample supply of milk. Rooming-in is recommended when the condition of the mother and infants permits it.

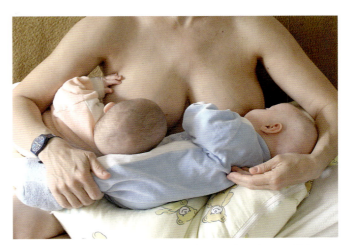

Fig. 47: A nursing pillow under the elbow makes the parallel position more comfortable [M307]

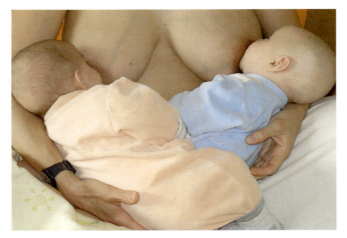

Fig. 48: The V position/cross-cradle position enables eye contact with both children [M307]

There are many possible positions in which to breastfeed twins simultaneously. Nevertheless, there are no general recommendations for simultaneous breastfeeding. Each mother must find out for herself and her infants, whether it is better for her to nurse one infant at a time or two at the same time. There can be times when one or more infants require more assistance with breastfeeding; then it is better to feed them individually. In any case, various positions for simultaneous breastfeeding should be shown and explained to the mother.

1.4 The older breastfed child

The World Health Organization (7) recommends exclusive breastfeeding for the first six months and subsequently the introduction of age-appropriate solid foods with the simultaneous continuation of breastfeeding at least until the second birthday and after that as long as desired by the mother and child. Most countries in Middle and Southern Europe, in contrast to Scandinavia, are currently still far from implementing this recommendation, which applies to *all* children around the world. (21) Therefore, the public is often astonished to see toddlers being breastfed. Only 23% of children in Australia for example are still being breastfed on their first birthday.*

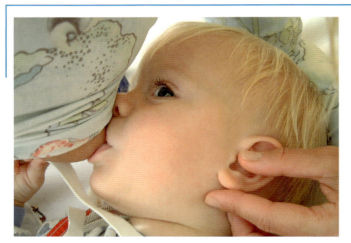

Fig. 49: Sick or unwell toddlers often have an increased need for breastfeeding, nursing gives security in a strange environment [M307]

Breastfeeding of older babies and toddlers differs from that of newborn infants.

The older the child, the less important the nutritional aspect of breastfeeding. Nevertheless, the health advantages of breastfeeding the child should not be underestimated. (22) There is no upper limit for the duration of breastfeeding and no evidence for harm with respect to psychology or development when breastfeeding continues into the third year of life or longer. (23) It is expected that the child will wean itself between the second and fourth birthday. (24)

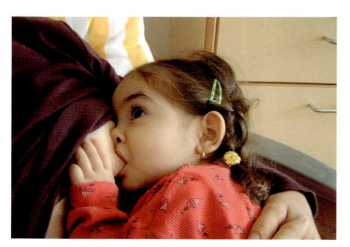

Fig. 50: Breastfeeding is still important even after the first birthday [M307]

* Breastfeeding in Australia, 2001 (Australian Bureau of Statistics, 2003) Online. Available: www.abs.gov.au/ausstats/abs@.nsf/cat/4810.0.55.001

1.5 Tandem breastfeeding

The older child is not always weaned before a new sibling is born. Unfortunately, many women are unnecessarily worried by the unproven statement that a new pregnancy makes immediate weaning necessary. However, no study has shown that breastfeeding in pregnancy is harmful to the unborn child. In the case of a normal pregnancy and a healthy mother, it is the decision of the woman alone whether to continue breastfeeding during the pregnancy. (25, 26)

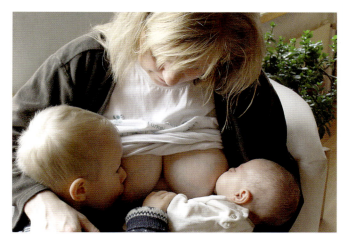

Fig. 51: The composition of breast milk adjusts itself for the youngest child [M307]

1.6 Appearance of breast milk

Breast milk clearly differs in appearance from the familiar sight of homogenised milk from cows. If breast milk is left to stand for a longer period, the milk fat separates out. Therefore, expressed breast milk should be carefully mixed before feeding to redistribute the milk fat again.

The colour of fresh breast milk varies between yellowish, bluish or even brownish. Frozen breast milk can take on a yellowish colour, which however does not mean that the milk is spoiled, unless it smells or tastes bad. When the lipase content is high, frozen breast milk can develop a soapy taste, which does not bother many children and is not harmful. (27) Food and medication can affect the colour of breast milk. Thus, there are reports of pink, orange, green and even black breast milk. This is, however, usually not a reason for concern. (28, 30)

1.6.1 Colostrum

At the start of the development of lactogenesis I around the 20th week of pregnancy, a colostrum-like fluid is first produced. Production of true colostrum begins subsequently in late pregnancy. Colostrum, which is yellowish to orange in appearance due to its high carotene content, has a high immunoglobulin level, acts as a laxative and thus can combat neonatal jaundice. In comparison to mature breast milk, colostrum contains less fat and carbohydrate, but more protein. Despite its very small quantity, colostrum supplies everything required by a newborn baby in the very first days. (31, 32)

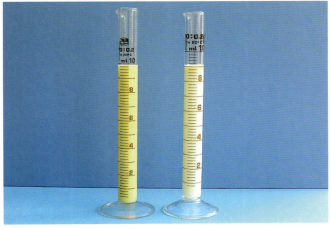

Fig. 52: Colostrum at 30 hours post partum from two different women [M307]

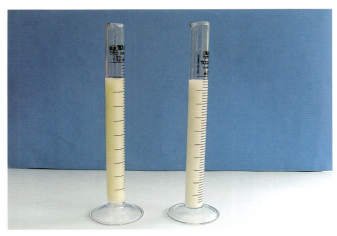

Fig. 53: Transitional milk at seven days post partum from two different mothers [M307]

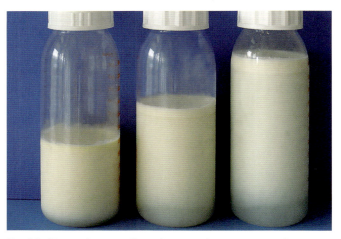

Fig. 54: Mature breast milk at three weeks post partum from three different mothers; the difference in fat content is clearly visible [M307]

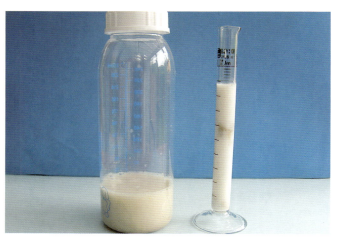

Fig. 55: Blood in breast milk without a visible injury to the nipple [M307]

1.6.2 Transitional milk

During the first four days postpartum, lactogenesis II begins, the so-called copious milk secretion. The initial coming-in of milk takes place in this phase. The changeover from colostrum to transitional milk cannot be determined exactly; the transition is fluent. There is an obvious increase in the content of lactose, fat and α-lactalbumin, while immunoglobulin levels and the total protein content fall. By the tenth day postpartum, approximately 50% of all mothers are producing mature breast milk. (📖 33, 34)

1.6.3 Mature breast milk

Just as there is no exact point in time that can be determined for the start of lactogenesis II, it is not possible either to establish exactly the end of this phase and the start of lactogenesis III (galactopoiesis). From the start of lactogenesis III, autocrine regulation of milk production predominates and the quantity of milk is adjusted according to the principle of supply and demand. (📖 31, 32) Mature breast milk can vary very greatly in colour and also the fat content can differ substantially not only from woman to woman, but even in the course of one breastfeed. (📖 35)

1.6.4 Blood in breast milk

Blood in breast milk can be due to various causes. Injured nipples (☞ 2.4) or an extended or increased vascularity and epithelial proliferation, for example due to the growth of the breast in pregnancy, are the most frequent reasons for blood in breast milk. It is essential that persistent bloody secretions from the breast are investigated by a doctor. As a rule, the blood does not harm the infant.

1.7 Elimination, stool and urine output in the newborn

1.7.1 Meconium

Meconium is the first stool of the newborn infant. It consists of shed intestinal epithelial cells, fatty substances, mucus, bile pigment, fermented digestion products as well as swallowed squamous epithelial cells and lanugo hairs. Meconium is almost odour-free and very sticky. Rapid elimination of the meconium is important. Delayed elimination can indicate a disease and can intensify neonatal jaundice due to the reabsorption of bilirubin. (☞ 2.6.13)

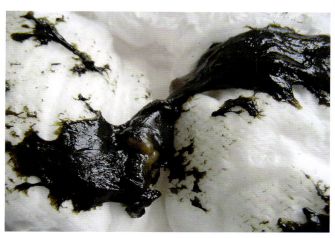

Fig. 56: The first bowel movement at five hours after birth [M307]

1.7.2 Transitional stools

As soon as the newborn infant receives breast milk (or a substitute product), the appearance of the stools changes: they become wetter, more liquid, less sticky and lighter. Transitional stools are a mixture of meconium and breast milk stools. A rapid elimination of meconium and the change to breast milk stools is an indication of a satisfactory intake of fluid and calories and decreases the risk of exacerbated neonatal jaundice. (📖 36, 37)

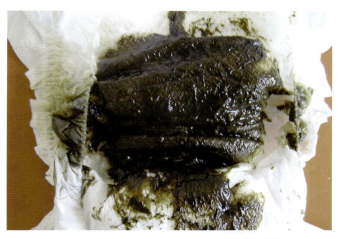

Fig. 57: Transitional stool at 24 hours after birth [M307]

1.7.3 Breast milk stools

After three to five days, the stools of the newborn infant should be yellow or yellowish-green in colour. After the first day of life, at least three bowel movements daily are to be expected. Less frequent bowel movements as well as the absence of a colour change are indications of inadequate milk intake, which must be investigated. (📖 38)

In the neonatal period, it is not unusual for stools to be excreted at each breastfeeding session.

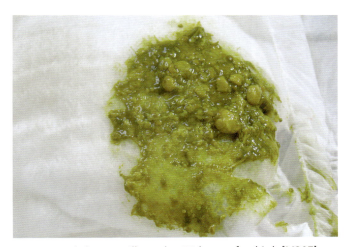

Fig. 58: Curdy breast milk stool at 30 hours after birth [M307]

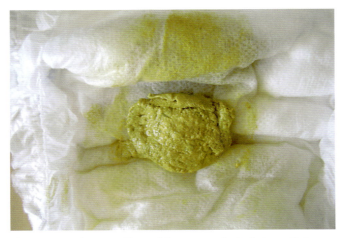

Fig. 59: Pasty breast milk stool from an exclusively breastfed infant at six days postpartum [M307]

As soon as the meconium has been totally eliminated, the stools of an exclusively breastfed baby are loose and unformed, often of a consistency similar to that of pea soup or cottage cheese. The colour can range from yellow to yellowish green to brownish. Occasionally, mucus may also be mixed in. The odour is bland and non-offensive.

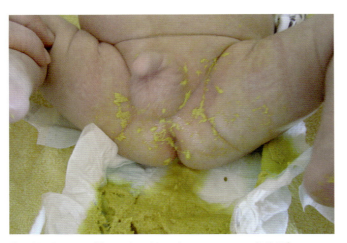

Fig. 60: Breast milk stool at 2 weeks post partum [M307]

Many breastfed infants have frequent bowel movements through the whole breastfeeding period. In others, the number of bowel movements decreases clearly after the first four to six weeks, with a corresponding increase in the quantity per stool. After the neonatal period, exclusively breastfed infants may have a bowel movement only once every five to seven days or even less frequently. These infrequent bowel movements should not be confused with constipation (hard, dry stools). Dry stools are an indication of inadequate milk intake.

1.7.4 Stools from formula fed infants

The stools of infants that are not breastfed are pale yellow to light brown in colour, frequently greenish if hypoallergenic formula is used. They have a stiffer, rubbery consistency and have a much more offensive odour than breast milk stools.

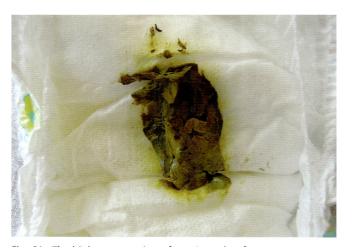

Fig. 61: The higher proportion of casein makes faeces more rubbery when formula milk is used [M307]

1.7.5 Bloody stools

Blood in the stool is a warning sign that should always be taken seriously. It can indicate necrotising enterocolitis (NEC), sepsis, coagulatory disorders, bowel obstruction or ischaemia as well as viral/bacterial intestinal infections with respiratory distress or fluid and electrolyte imbalances. To a certain extent, blood admixed with stool can indicate an allergic reaction or an intolerance to food eaten by the mother/child. (📖 39)

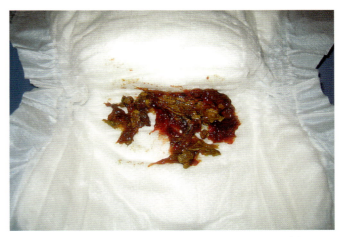

Fig. 62: Blood in the stools should always be investigated: here suspected NEC in a 6-day-old baby born at 37 weeks' gestation [O448]

1.7.6 Urine

Brick-dust sediment
Especially in the very first days postpartum, this red urinary sediment may be found in the nappy of the newborn infant. Due to their appearance, these urinary crystals are called brick-dust sediment. They can be an indication of reduced fluid intake. From the fourth day onwards, an exclusively breastfed infant should have at least six wet nappies per day (24 h).

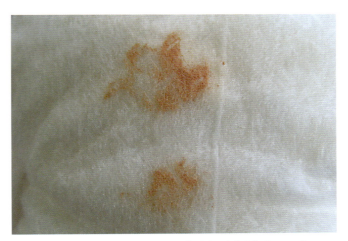

Fig. 63: Often mistaken by parents for blood: brick-dust sediment [M307]

2
Breastfeeding problems and their causes

2.1 Atypical breast shapes 26

2.2. Problematic nipple forms 30

2.3 Pathological changes of the breast 34

2.4. Pain and injury of the nipple 37

2.5 Lifestyle 41

2.6 Infants with special needs 42

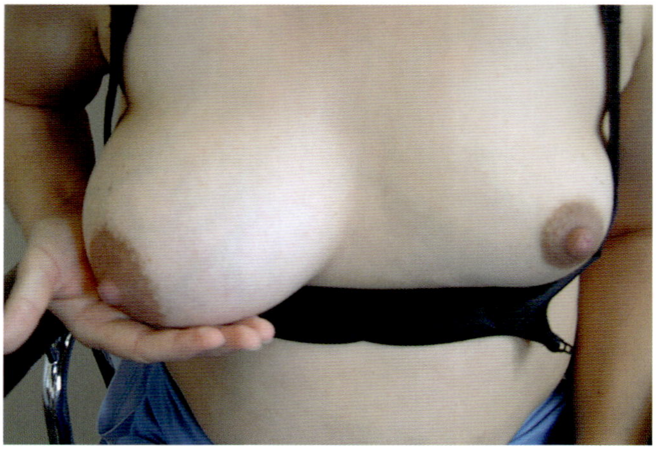

2.1 Atypical breast shapes

2.1.1 Asymmetric breasts

Sufficient mammary gland tissue
No woman has breasts of absolutely the same size. However, already before and during pregnancy, breasts that clearly differ in size can be an indication of insufficient mammary gland tissue and thus of future problems with breastfeeding. If one breast is unable to produce milk, or not produce it optimally, the woman can generally feed from the other breast, if sufficient mammary gland tissue is present. Women with small breasts may have to breastfeed more frequently, since their breasts have a smaller storage capacity. (☞ 40–42)

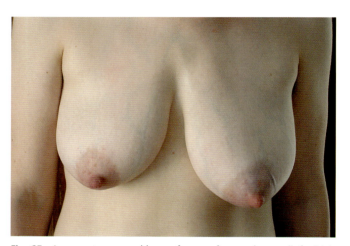

Fig. 64: Asymmetric but sufficient glandular tissue. The mother breastfed for several months (both breasts) [M307]

Asymmetry due to preference for one breast
Occasionally there will be asymmetric development of the breasts during lactation, because the infant suckles more frequently or more efficiently from one side or because the mother preferentially nurses on one side. When the child is thriving, this development is, if anything, a cosmetic problem that will even out again after weaning (☞ Fig. 14).

Fig. 65: Asymmetry caused by preference for one breast (left side) at nine weeks postpartum [M307]

2.1.2 Inadequate mammary gland tissue

Tubular breasts
Rees and Aston describe the characteristics of tubular (tuberous) breasts in the following way: small breast base, short vertical extent of glandular tissue, large areola, frequent pseudoherniation of the mammary gland tissue in the areola, hypoplasia of the lower quadrants, nipple dysplasia and obligate anomalies of the maternal hand such as brachydactyly, oligodactyly or syndactyly. The inadequate development of the mammary gland tissue in women with this anomaly frequently means that breastfeeding (fully) is not possible. (☞ 43)

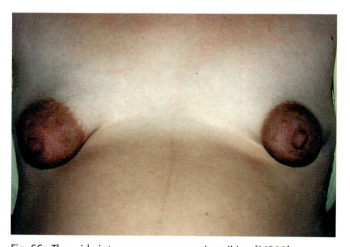

Fig. 66: The wide intramammary space is striking [M308]

Poland's syndrome

Poland's syndrome (Amazon syndrome) is a congenital, usually unilateral malformation of the mammary glands and breast muscles as well as of the skin and appendages, in which malformations of the ribs and hands may also occur. (📖 44) Women with Poland's syndrome have one healthy and one underdeveloped or missing breast. The ability to breastfeed from the unaffected breast is usually normal.

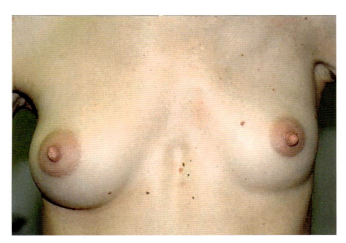

Fig. 67: The pectoralis major muscle is missing on the left [T346]

2.1.3 Accessory mammary gland tissue

The milk line, from which the milk glands develop, extends from the axilla to the groin. Occasionally, during the embryonic period, there is incomplete involution of the milk line, as a consequence of which supernumerary nipples and accessory mammary tissue develop. This ectopic mammary gland tissue can develop more or less predominant, being especially frequent in the area between the breast and the arm pit. In rare cases, complete supernumerary (accessory) mammary glands may develop (polymastia). (📖 45)

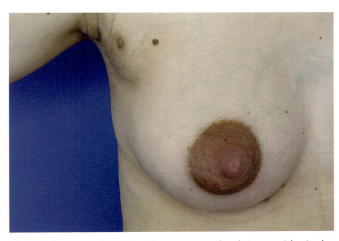

Fig. 68: Accessory (additional) mammary gland tissue with nipple in the axilla [M307]

Ectopic mammary gland tissue is also subject to hormone-dependent development and cycles. Thus it is mostly first discovered in puberty or during pregnancy. It may not only be cosmetically disturbing, but can also cause problems. Tumours may also develop in accessory mammary gland tissue. (📖 46)

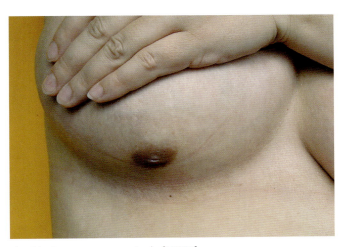

Fig. 69: Supernumerary nipple [M307]

2.1 Atypical breast shapes

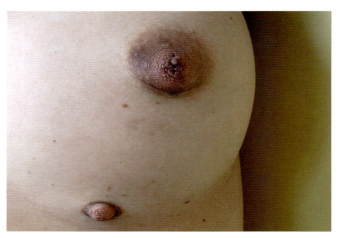

Fig. 70: Fully developed supernumerary nipple with a small areola [M307]

While accessory mammary gland tissue is relatively rare, supernumerary nipples occur much more frequently. Accessory nipples (polythelia) appear exclusively along the milk line. Not infrequently, they are mistaken for moles, warts or even skin tumours. Supernumerary nipples can appear in both women and men and have no pathological significance. Removal may be desired for cosmetic reasons.

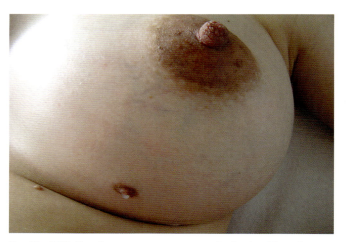

Fig. 71: Milk flow from a supernumerary nipple should not be stimulated [M307]

Accessory mammary gland tissue is not a reason for primary weaning. Milk production is possible in the accessory mammary gland tissue, which can lead to painful engorgement if there is no patent opening. The affected sites can be cooled and it is appropriate to use an analgesic compatible with breastfeeding, if required. Due to the lack of stimulation, milk production finally stops and usually no further problems occur.

2.1.4 Following breast surgery

In the past, women who had previously undergone breast surgery were mostly advised not to breastfeed. In many cases it was seldom possible for a women who had undergone breast surgery to breastfeed (fully) any more. Presently, improved surgical techniques mean that at least partial breastfeeding is often possible. As long as only one breast has undergone surgery, feeding with the unaffected breast is always possible.

Following surgery, there are three scenarios for how breastfeeding proceeds:
- Breastfeeding proceeds normally, because a minimal amount of milk ducts or large nerves have been severed or injured to cause a discernible difference in the quantity of milk received by the infant. Or the milk ducts have regrown after the injury.
- During the first six weeks, the infant gains weight well, because the elevated maternal hormone levels lead to additional milk production. Then the infant's weight gain slows down and supplementary feeding becomes necessary.
- The maternal milk production is low from the start and must be supplemented at an early stage. The infant can continue to be breastfed for as long as the mother and child wish.

The general advice should be to postpone cosmetic breast surgery until family planning is complete. (✎ 47)

Breast enlargement (augmentation)
The initial size of the breasts and the types of incisions during surgery are important for conserving the ability to breastfeed. If the incisions are in the submammary fold or near the axilla, it can be assumed that the implant was placed behind the milk ducts and that these and also the larger nerves have therefore not been injured. In this case, the ability to breastfeed should not be affected. However, scar tissue develops in the breast as a response to breast augmentation, and this may possibly lead to pain and discomfort during breastfeeding, especially during lactogenesis II. (📖 47)

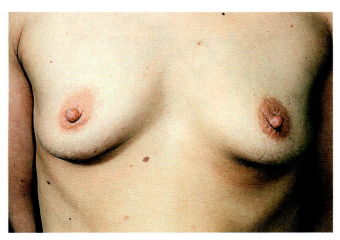

Fig. 72: Before breast enlargement [T347]

If a flexible implant is used, it is important to discuss correct attachment in detail with the mother and to observe several breastfeeds because a good latch is often difficult with a moveable implant. If production problems with the milk occur in women following breast augmentation, it should always be taken into consideration that the reason for considering the breast to be small before the augmentation could have been due to insufficient mammary gland tissue. (📖 47)

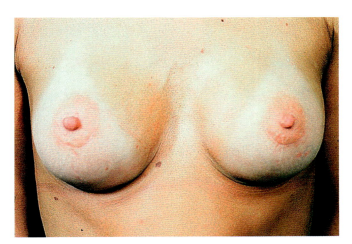

Fig. 73: After breast enlargement [T347]

Breast reduction
During breast reduction, part of the breast tissue is removed. In this case, the milk ducts are nearly always severed and the nerves damaged. Occasionally, the nipple is removed and replaced in another location. The more breast tissue removed, the smaller the chance a woman can (fully) breastfeed her infant after breast surgery. If the nipple has been relocated, the chance is reduced even further. However, there are reports of women in whom milk ducts and also nerves have grown together again. (📖 47)

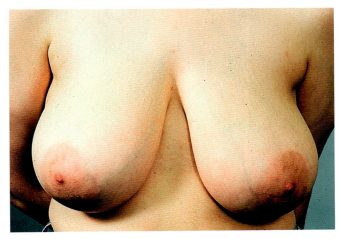

Fig. 74: Before breast reduction [T347]

2.1 Atypical breast shapes

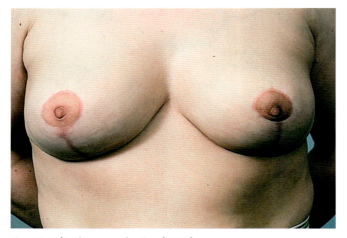

Fig. 75: After breast reduction [T347]

Some women fear that breastfeeding could affect the cosmetic result of the surgery. These women should know that changes to the breasts are primarily due to pregnancy and not to lactation (☞ Fig. 14). Following weaning, the glandular tissue recedes and is replaced by fatty tissue. In most cases, some time after weaning, the breast regains its normal appearance, so that, in the long term, the cosmetic result of the breast reduction is not affected. The process can take up to three years. (📖 47)

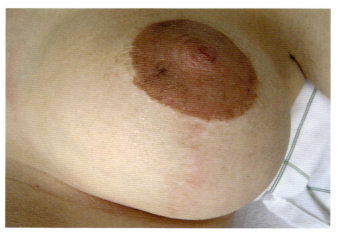

Fig. 76: Full breastfeeding was possible for several months two years after removal of 500 g breast tissue from the left breast and 975 g from the right breast [M307]

Engorgement may occur after the birth due to the scarring, which cannot be resolved by means of breastfeeding, because the milk ducts have been so damaged that emptying is no longer possible. In this case, failure of the breast to be emptied in this region causes atrophy due to pressure in the affected milk ducts.

Milk production ceases and the congestion resolves. In between breastfeeding, the breast can be cooled and, when required, an analgesic compatible with breastfeeding can be used. (📖 47)

2.2 Problematic nipple forms

2.2.1 Flat nipples

Infants are attached to the breast and not to the nipple. If the infant can latch onto the breast well, the shape of the nipple has a subordinate role. Flat nipples need not necessarily cause problems with breastfeeding. In many cases, flat nipples will often protrude with the appropriate stimulation. Correct attachment of and sucking by the child is of prime importance.

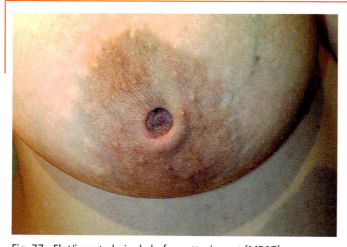

Fig. 77: Flat/inverted nipple before attachment [M307]

A well attached child will also stimulate and empty the breast when the nipples are flat, so that neither problems with sore nipples nor with the quantity of milk should be expected. If the nipples become flattened on account of overfull, taut breasts, it is helpful to express or carefully pump enough milk before the feed to make the breast and areola softer and easier for the infant to latch on. Early and frequent breastfeeds helps the infant to learn correct attachment and sucking before the initial coming-in of milk makes it more difficult to latch onto the breast.

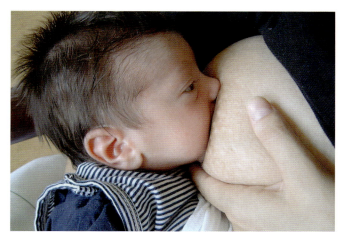

Fig. 78: Well attached child, well supported breast [M307]

Immediately after breastfeeding, flat nipples often remain protruded for some time. Mothers sometimes report that their nipples, which were flat before pregnancy or childbirth, become permanently protruded after a longer lactation period. The mother pictured was able to breastfeed two children exclusively for an extended time. Before breastfeeds, she first had to manually stimulate the nipples. Figures 77, 78 and 79 show the same mother.

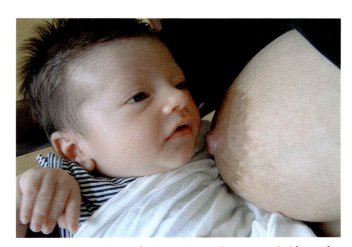

Fig. 79: Following breastfeeding, the nipple is protruded [M307]

2.2.2 Retracted/inverted nipples

Women can have one or both nipples inverted. In order to establish whether a nipple is actually inverted, the so-called 'pinch test' can be used. The areola is gently squeezed together about 2.5 cm behind the tip of the nipple. If the nipple then protrudes out, it is not a true inverted nipple and special treatment is not usually necessary. If the nipple draws back or takes on a concave curvature, it is an inverted nipple. Figures 80–83 show the same woman.

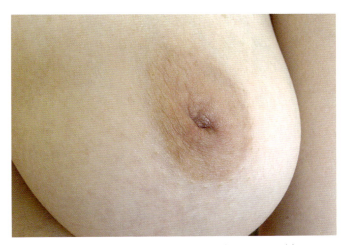

Fig. 80: Inverted nipple on the left breast of a 23-year-old woman, who has so far not been pregnant [M307]

2.2 Problematic nipple forms

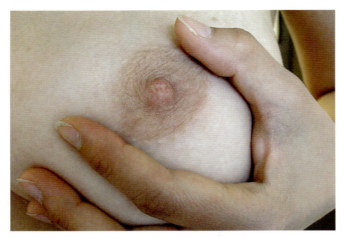

Fig. 81: Inverted left nipple after manual stimulation: breastfeeding problems are very unlikely [M307]

In the case of inverted nipples, the use of breast shells is often recommended during pregnancy in order to prepare for breastfeeding. Breast shells are supposed to cause nipple protrusion by means of constant pressure and exploitation of the increased tissue elasticity brought about by pregnancy. However, the efficacy of this breastfeeding aid is disputed. A newer aid for correction of inverted nipples is the Niplette (☞ 3.2.3). In the authors' experience, many women find the Niplette to be uncomfortable.

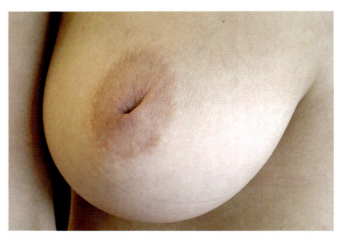

Fig. 82: Inverted nipple on the right breast [M307]

Following the birth, when necessary, a milk pump or other suction apparatus (☞ 3.2.3) can help to draw out flat or inverted nipples immediately before breastfeeding and thus make it easier for the infant to latch onto the breast.

In rare cases, the inversion of a nipple can lead to a reduction in the stimulation necessary to initiate sufficient prolactin release. As a result, there may be insufficient milk synthesis. (📖 48)

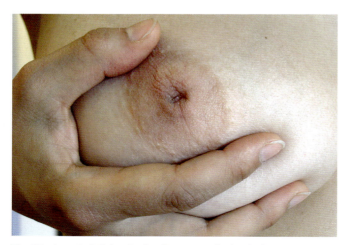

Fig. 83: Inverted right nipple after manual stimulation: breastfeeding problems are likely [M307]

Nipple shields (☞ 3.2.4) should never be offered as a first-line resource in the case of inverted nipples. Because the infant feeds at the breast and not at the nipple, the first step is to train the mother in correct attachment technique. Only when all other possibilities have been exhausted, should a nipple shield be used.

In the presence of inverted nipples, finger feeding is not recommended, because the finger can be a deterring stimulus for the child.

2.2.3 Small nipples

As a rule, small nipples do not present any problems for breastfeeding. Since the infant is not attached to the nipple but to the breast, and since as much breast tissue as possible in addition to the nipple should be taken into the mouth, the basic rule applies: attention should be given to optimal attachment and sucking.

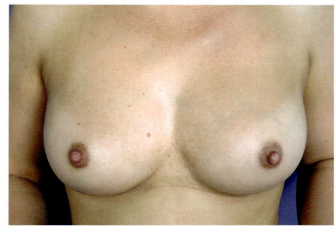

Fig. 84: Small nipples with a small areola: successful breastfeeding of a premature baby was possible [M307]

2.2.4 Large nipples

Large nipples may cause breastfeeding problems primarily in small infants with small mouths. If the infant is unable to take the nipple plus part of the areola fully into its mouth, this can lead to soreness and, on account of insufficient stimulation, to an inadequate milk supply. In occasional cases, nipple shields or milk expression can be a (temporary) solution.

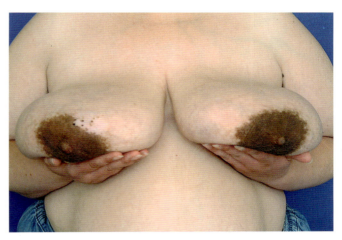

Fig. 85: Large nipples with a large areola and pigmentation disorder: successful breastfeeding was possible [M307]

2.2.5 Bifurcated or double nipples

A bifurcated nipple with a normally located areola is not necessarily a hindrance to breastfeeding. Nursing the infant should be attempted in such a way that the largest diameter of the nipple lies between the corners of the child's mouth. A discrepancy between the child's mouth and the size of the nipple causes problems.

There are cases in which attachment may not be possible and, instead, milk will need to be expressed. When expressing milk with a pump, attention must be paid to ensuring that the flange diameter corresponds to that of the nipple.

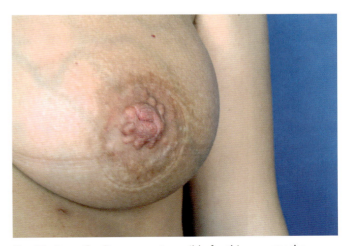

Fig. 86: Breastfeeding was not possible for this woman; the quantity of milk remained small [M307]

2.2 Problematic nipple forms

2.3 Pathological changes of the breast

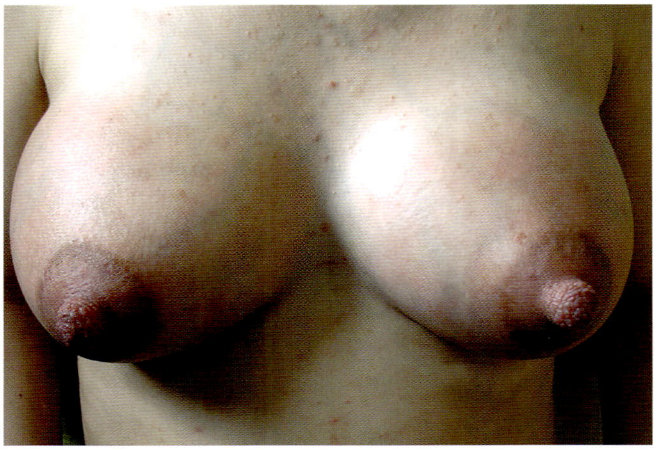

2.3.1 Mammary gland swelling (initial engorgement)

The cause of pathological mammary gland swelling is nearly always correlated with initial delayed attachment following delivery, infrequent nursing or time-limited duration of nursing. General engorgement can be limited to the breast itself (peripheral mammary gland swelling) and/or also to the areola. In areolar engorgement, the nipple is flattened so that it is difficult for the infant to latch onto it and the breast is no longer emptied efficiently.

Fig. 87: Extreme engorgement during Lactogenesis II [M307]

Insufficient emptying of the breast aggravates the engorgement. If the infant can no longer suck well at the taut breast, it is useful to express manually or with a pump, in order to make the areola softer and easier to latch onto. Treatment of choice involves frequent nursing around the clock, warm compresses before breastfeeding and cool ones afterwards, as well as the use of analgesics compatible with breastfeeding, as required. Lymphatic drainage and deep tissue massage may also be used.

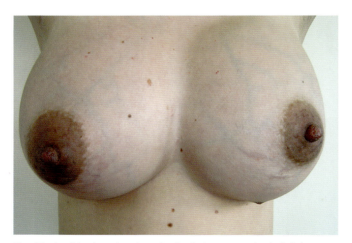

Fig. 88: In this situation, lymphatic drainage can be helpful [M307]

2.3.2 Local engorgement (plugged ducts)

Local engorgement occurs when one or more milk ducts are not emptied. The breast is often swollen (oedematous) and tender. In many cases, engorgement develops due to incorrect management of breastfeeding, but other causes such as restrictive clothing or pressure on the breast from a baby sling can prevent milk from flowing and cause stasis. Stress also seems to promote the development of stasis. Frequent nursing or expressing milk to empty the breast is the therapy of choice.

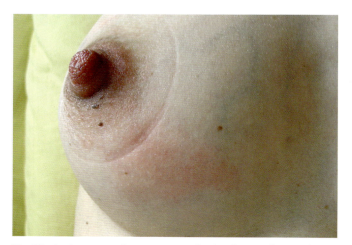

Fig. 89: In the event of engorgement lasting longer than 24 hours or with additional symptoms, medical investigation is required [M307]

2.3.3 Mastitis

Mastitis is an inflammation of the mammary gland tissue that can either be infectious or non-infectious. Mastitis is frequently preceded by milk stasis. The transition between engorgement and mastitis is not easily defined. As a rule, weaning is counterproductive, as continuation of breastfeeding promotes recovery. Therapy consists of frequent emptying of the breast, rest, cooling after breastfeeding and antibiotics, if required. If there is no improvement after 24 hours of conservative treatment, with continuation of fever, headache or flu-like symptoms in the limbs, medical investigation is imperative. The main cause of mastitis is the mother being overburdened!

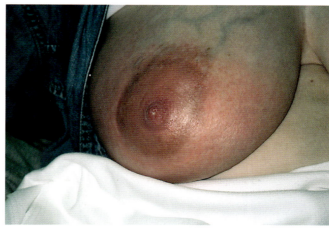

Fig. 90: Frequent breastfeeding and rest are essential in the treatment of mastitis [M307]

2.3.4 Abscess

If an abscess develops during the course of mastitis, it must be drained, either by surgical incision or by ultrasound-guided needle or catheter aspiration or drainage. During surgery, the direction of the incision should be chosen so as to make continued breastfeeding or the re-initiation of breastfeeding possible. The incision should be made as far as possible from the areola, however there should not be too great a distance between the site of puncture and the abscess, in order to minimise the potential risk of bacterial spread. (☞ 49)

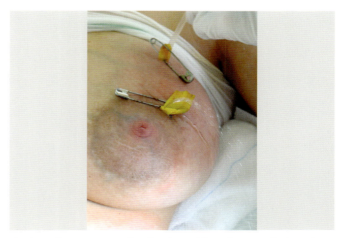

Fig. 91: Abscesses can also develop without fever and when the quantity of milk is small [M307]

During breastfeeding, the wound should be dressed so that the child does not come into contact with the wound or secretions from it. If attaching the child is too painful for the mother, careful manual expression or pumping must be used to prevent stasis. Milk can trickle from the incision over an extended period, however this does not promote increased fistula development or other complications. Figures 91 and 92 show the same woman.

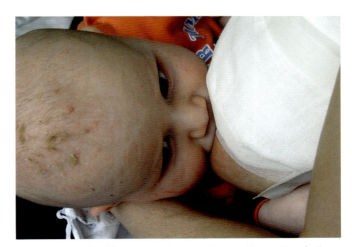

Fig. 92: Breastfeeding can continue as long as the mother feels able to do so (wound covered with dressing) [M307]

2.3 Pathological changes of the breast

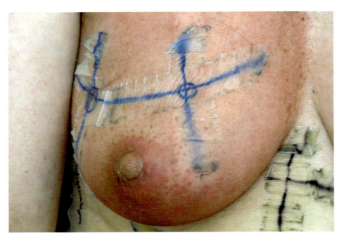

Fig. 93: Breast during radiation therapy [M307]

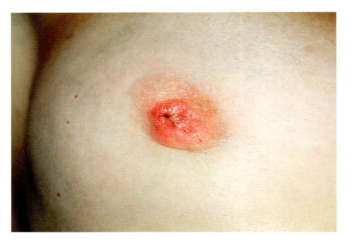

Fig. 94: Nipple cancer [T346]

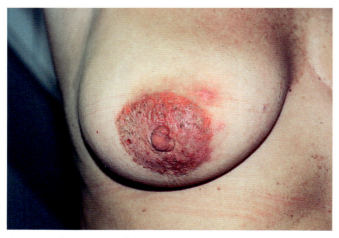

Fig. 95: Inflammation of the nipple should not be confused with nipple cancer [T346]

2.3.5 Breast cancer

Current research indicates that approximately 1 in 11 women will be diagnosed with breast cancer before age 75.* If cancer is diagnosed during lactation, weaning is necessary. Whether breastfeeding is still possible after therapy depends on the extent of damage to the breasts. According to a study from 2002, breastfeeding has a protective effect against breast cancer. (📖 50, 51)

2.3.6 Nipple cancer (Paget's disease of the nipple)

Nipple cancer, or Paget's disease of the nipple, is a specific form of ductal carcinoma in situ, in which the carcinoma infiltrates the nipple and the surrounding skin. Paget's disease of the nipple is thought to account for 1%–4% of all cases of breast cancer. Symptoms include itching, burning sensation, redness and flaking of the skin from the nipples and areola and possibly also bloody secretion from the nipple.

Eczema and inflammation of the nipples that do not respond to treatment could be a symptom of Paget's disease of the nipple. Thus a careful medical investigation by a dermatologist is necessary if a nipple condition does not heal successfully. (📖 52)

* Breast Cancer in Australia: An Overview, 2006 (Australian Institute of Health and Welfare and National Breast Cancer Centre, 2006) Online. Available: www.nbcc.org.au/best-practice/resources/BCR_breastcancerinaustra.pdf

2.4 Pain and injury of the nipple

2.4.1 Sore nipples

Sore nipples is one of the most frequent reasons for early weaning. In the first few days following the delivery, the nipples may be somewhat sensitive, but anything over and above this sensitivity is not normal. Painful breastfeeding is a reason to examine attachment technique and sucking behaviour; also inspect the mouth of the infant (lingual frenulum). Nipple shields, ointments and tinctures do not solve the problem and may even delay healing.

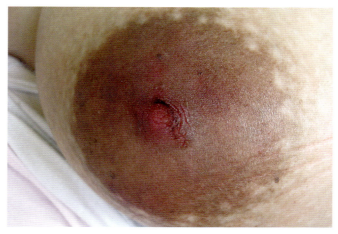

Fig. 96: The causes of sore nipples must be found and eliminated [M307]

2.4.2 Nipple fissures

Open nipple wounds are an entry point for pathogens of all types, which can lead to mastitis. It is useful to nurse the infant in such a way that the open wound lies exactly at the corner of its mouth. This decreases stress on the wound during breastfeeding. In particularly bad cases, a temporary interruption of breastfeeding can be useful, during which the milk is expressed manually or with the careful use of an efficient pump. During the breastfeeding pause an alternative feeding method should be chosen (☞ 3.3).

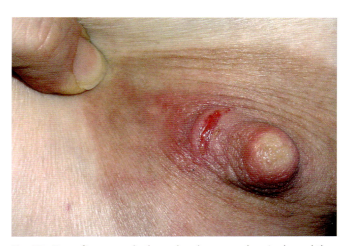

Fig. 97: Deep fissure at the boundary between the nipple and the areola with additional vasospasm [O446]

To avoid nipple injury, it is important to correctly remove the infant from the breast when it does not release the breast spontaneously. First the sucking seal must be released. To do this, a finger can be inserted carefully into the corner of the infant's mouth and downward pressure applied to the lower jaw in order to break the seal. The nipple must never be pulled from the child's mouth without releasing the sucking seal.

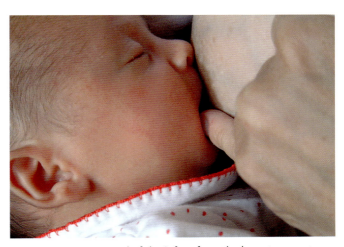

Fig. 98: Correct removal of the infant from the breast prevents nipple injury [M307]

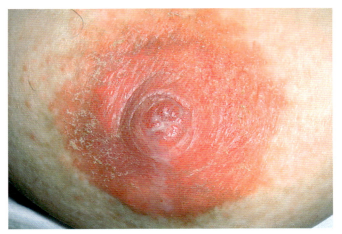

Fig. 99: Pronounced candidiasis with additional bacterial infection [M308]

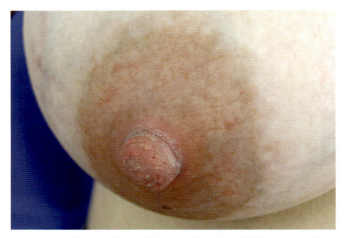

Fig. 100: Mild case of candidiasis with a whitish film; the mother experienced very severe pain [M307]

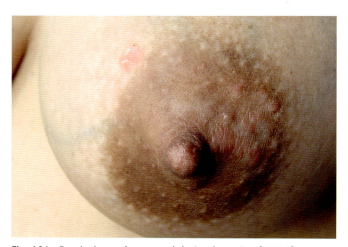

Fig. 101: Psoriasis can be treated during lactation [M307]

2.4.3 *Candida*/thrush

Candida albicans is the commensal organism that causes oral thrush as well as yeast infections of the vagina, is a fungus that thrives in a damp, dark environment, for example, on the nipples, in the milk ducts and in the vagina of the mother, and in the mouth and nappy area of the baby. Candidiasis of the nipples can be extremely painful. It requires rigorous treatment of the mother *and* child with antifungal medication, even when the baby appears to be asymptomatic. The treatment should continue for several days after the symptoms have resolved. (✎ 53)

After each breastfeeding session, the nipples are rinsed with clear water. This serves to remove milk residues in order to deprive the *Candida* of its growth medium. Breast milk residues must never be allowed to dry on the breast! Until the pain subsides, it can be useful to shorten the breastfeeding sessions and instead nurse more frequently. In extreme cases, it can be useful to interrupt breastfeeding for a period. Since the pain usually subsides as soon as the milk ejection reflex (☞ 1.2.3) starts, it is advisable to begin breastfeeding with the less painful breast. Absolute hygiene is essential. *Candida* is not inactivated by freezing!

2.4.4 Psoriasis

Psoriasis is an autoimmune disease that occurs in the form of flare ups and can appear on any part of the body, including the breast, areola and nipple. The experience of some women is that the breasts and nipples are only affected during lactation. Psoriasis can make breastfeeding very painful, so that interruption of breastfeeding is necessary, and even weaning in extreme cases. Local treatment with corticosteroids is possible during lactation.

2.4.5 Allergic reactions

Allergic reactions or intolerance can occur at any time, although women seem to be more at risk after giving birth. Frequent triggers for allergic skin reactions on the breasts are detergents, soaps, shower gels and other toiletries and cosmetics as well as breast ointments and medicinal products. Reactions to the component material of nipple shields, breast shells and flanges of breast pumps have also been reported.

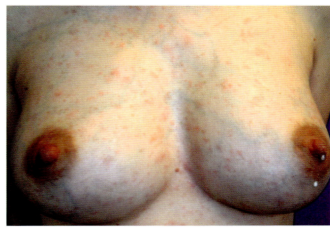

Fig. 102: Allergic reaction to antibiotics prescribed for mastitis [M307]

Residues of supplementary food in the mouth of the child, or traces of solid food or drink transferred in the child's saliva can also result in allergic reactions of the breasts and nipples. There have also been occasional reports that the changes in composition of a child's saliva during teething can result in allergic skin reactions.

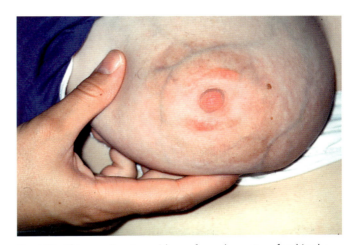

Fig. 103: Skin reaction to residues of supplementary food in the child's mouth [M307]

2.4.6 Virus infections – Herpes

Herpes simplex I (oral) and II (genital) are viruses transmitted through contact with active lesions. When herpes occurs on the breast or nipple, there is a risk that the infant will become infected, which can be life-threatening. It is essential to prevent the infant coming into contact with the active lesions. Milk should be expressed from the affected breast and discarded until the lesions have healed. Likewise, in the case of oral herpes (e.g. in the mother, caregiver), contact with the lesions should be prevented (e.g. no kissing the infant).

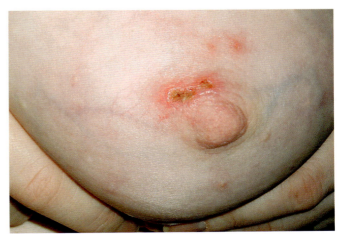

Fig. 104: Herpes is only a contraindication to breastfeeding when either breast is affected [O447]

2.4 Pain and injury of the nipple

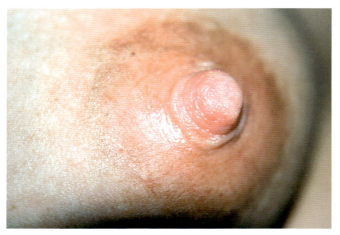

Fig. 105: The ischaemic nipple is an indication of vasospasm [O445]

2.4.7 Raynaud's phenomenon/vasospasm

During vasospasm of the nipple, the blood flow to the nipple is occasionally affected. The nipple becomes white and numb. As soon as the blood circulates normally again, the colour of the nipple changes rapidly to bluish and then becomes red. The return of the flow of blood is associated with severe pain, which can continue for a variable period. Triggers include cold, stress and some medications. In recent years, nipple vasospasm has increasingly been observed in women that have taken high-dose magnesium shortly before giving birth. (📖 54)

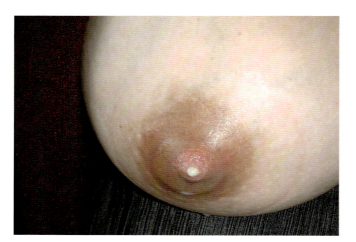

Fig. 106: Frequently occurring milk blisters can indicate that the mother is overburdened [M308]

2.4.8 Milk bleb/milk blisters

Milk blebs can arise due to a plug of thickened milk, which obstructs milk flow from a nipple pore. Occasionally, a thin piece of skin can also hamper the flow of the milk. This can lead to stasis and pain if the blockage is not removed. Warm, damp compresses and subsequent nursing of the child generally suffice to open the blister and relieve the engorgement. Occasionally, a milk blister has to be opened by a doctor using a sterile needle.

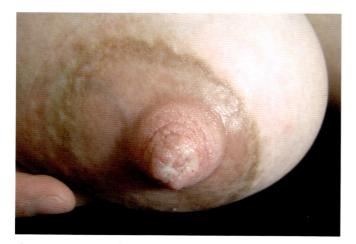

Fig. 107: Bacterial infection of the nipple [M307]

2.4.9 Bacterial infections

Bacterial infections of the nipple can occur in any phase of lactation. Skin that has been previously damaged is particularly at risk. Bacterial infections can be extremely painful and occasionally require breastfeeding to be interrupted and the milk to be expressed. Treatment is usually topical, with an antibacterial ointment or cream. Systemic treatment is rarely necessary.

2.5 Lifestyle

2.5.1 Tattoos

In recent years, tattoos have become increasingly more popular and thus breastfeeding counsellors come across women with breast tattoos more frequently. Tattoos have no impact on breastfeeding. Nevertheless, it would be advisable to refrain from obtaining tattoos during the lactation period. Although the possibility that ink could pass into the breast milk is small, there is a risk of infection with human immunodefiency virus (HIV), hepatitis B and C as well as other infectious diseases.

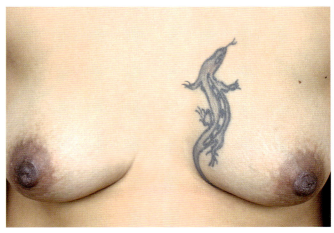

Fig. 108: Tattoo on a non-lactating breast [M307]

Milk banks often ask whether a potential donor has been tattooed or pierced in the preceding six or twelve months. On safety grounds, milk from women who have been tattooed or pierced within this period is refused by milk banks. (55)

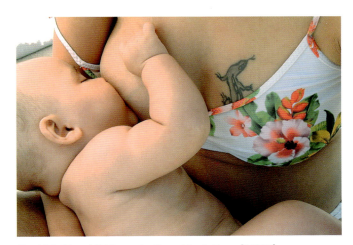

Fig. 109: The child is not bothered by tattoos [M307]

2.5.2 Piercing

In most cases, nipple piercing does not cause any problems with breastfeeding. The jewellery must be removed when breastfeeding, because there is a risk that it could injure or be swallowed by the child. Removal of the jewellery for breastfeeding is also advisable for hygienic reasons. There are reports of cases where, due to piercing jewellery being worn in the nipple, milk leakage has occurred from the breast of women who have previously not been pregnant. (56)

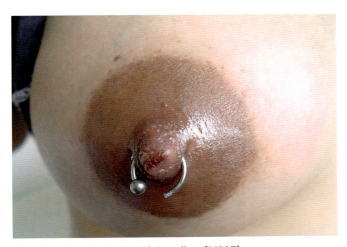

Fig. 110: Pierced nipple with jewellery [M307]

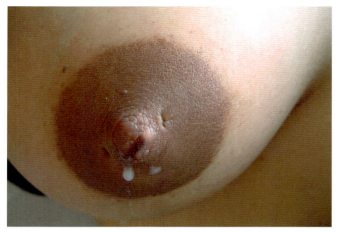

Fig. 111: Pierced nipple: the fissure was caused by incorrect attachment [M307]

If the piercing jewellery is permanently removed during the lactation period, the hole can grow over and will have to be pierced again following the end of lactation, if a piercing is still desired at that time. If the jewellery is removed for each breastfeeding session, the hole will remain patent, but the constant insertion and removal of the jewellery can result in soreness and thus in problems with breastfeeding.

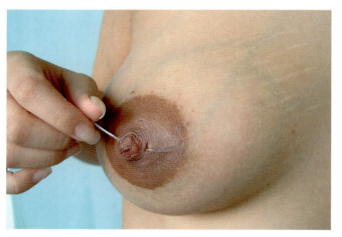

Fig. 112: Daily use of a plastic bar to keep the pierced channel patent [M307]

Some women prefer not to insert any jewellery during the lactation period and regularly use a bar made of PMFP (polyethylene medical flexible plastic) to keep the pierced channel patent. It is not known whether this method results in less irritation than the regular insertion of jewellery. Figures 110, 111 and 112 each show the same mother.

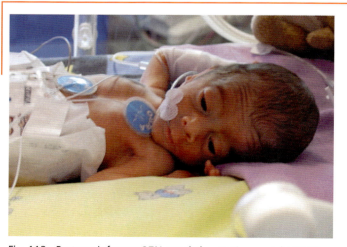

Fig. 113: Preterm infant at 27 1/7 weeks' gestation, weight 1140 g [M307]

2.6 Infants with special needs

2.6.1 Prematurity

A preterm delivery is when the infant is born before the end of the 37th week of gestation. Premature infants are classified into those with low birth weight (LBW, less than 2500 g), very low birth weight (VLBW, birth usually before the end of the 32nd week of gestation, weight less than 1500 g), as well as infants with extremely low birth weight (ELBW, birth before the end of the 28th week of gestation, weight less than 1000 g). The individual weights can vary between the 10th and 90th percentiles. (📖 57)

In comparison to the 1970s and 1980s, the mortality of premature babies has been drastically reduced worldwide due to progress in perinatal medicine and the experience of professionals in the field. Factors central to this progress include the antenatal use of steroids and improved perinatal care. In addition, developments in respirator support, such as CPAP (continuous positive airway pressure) and the administration of surfactant to an increasing number of preterm infants, improves outcomes.

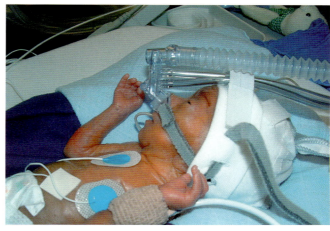

Fig. 114: Extremely small preterm infant with CPAP, born at $25^{5/7}$ weeks' gestation, weight 630 g [O448]

For mothers with premature or sick newborn infants, expressing milk via a breast pump and feeding via a tube is often the only alternative to breastfeeding until the infant is sufficiently developed to be able to be fed orally. In this situation, the mother has a unique role: she is the only person who can provide her milk for her infant. (📖 58)

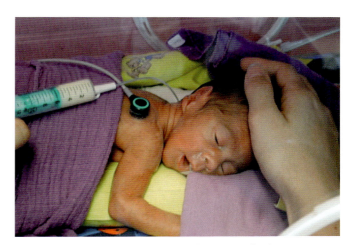

Fig. 115: Intubated, small preterm infant; bolus feeding is associated with a better weight gain (📖 59) [M307]

It has been reported that the optimal time frame to commence expressing milk is within the first six hours following delivery. (📖 60) After a premature delivery, the commencement of lactation can be delayed or affected in some women. The reasons for this are not fully understood. However, it is not a question of a lack of prolactin. (📖 41, 61) An indication of long-term inadequate milk production is the mother producing less than 500 mL of milk per day at the end of the second week postpartum. (📖 62)

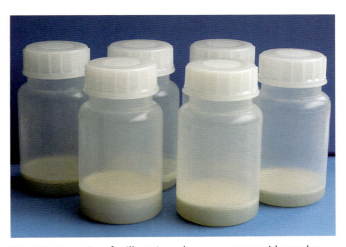

Fig. 116: Quantity of milk at 4 weeks post partum with regular milk expression over 24 hours [M307]

2.6 Infants with special needs

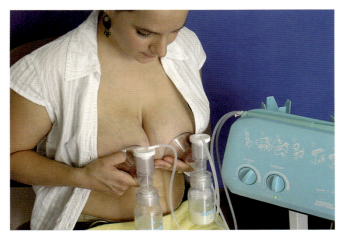

Fig. 117: Dual expression saves time and promotes milk synthesis [M307]

The release of prolactin is essential for milk synthesis. (👉 41) This release is regulated by stimulation. The total duration of pumping required over 24 hours for a mother to achieve an optimal supply of milk is approximately 100 minutes. (👉 63) Short and frequent expressing is recommended over longer expression times with long intervals in between. For optimal results, dual expression with a fully automatic, electric hospital grade pump is recommended. (👉 62, 91)

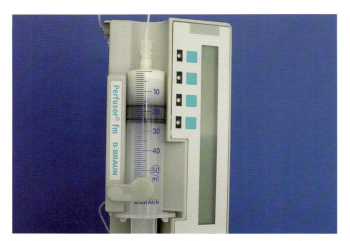

Fig. 118: Feeding tube plus syringe placed in a pump positioned vertically; the milk fat has settled at the top [M307]

The preterm infant receives most of its energy from the fat in breast milk. Continuous tube feeding results in a greater loss of fat, because the milk fat sticks to the tubing compared with intermittent tube feeding with a defined bolus. The longer the tube and the longer the duration of feeding, the more fat will be lost. If continuous feeding is indicated, the fat loss can be reduced from 48% to 8% if a pump system is used, in which the point of the syringe is directed upwards. (👉 64)

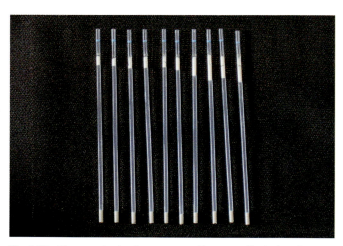

Fig. 119: Changes in the fat content of breast milk during the course of expression (👉 35) [O449]

The milk samples in Fig. 119 were obtained by expressing at one-minute intervals. They were then drawn up into capillary tubes, sealed at the bottom end, and then centrifuged. The milk fat is clearly recognisable as a white layer over the clear, skimmed milk. The ratio of the length of the fat column to that of the total milk column in the capillary tubes expressed as a percentage gives the creamatocrit value. This value enables the energy content of the milk to be calculated. The sample on the left shows a low creamatocrit, which increases in samples to the right in proportion to the degree of emptying of the breast.

More and more human milk banks are being set up around the world to supply preterm infants, sick newborn infants and also older recipients (e.g. those under treatment for cancer) with milk from donors. Preterm infants profit from donor milk when their own mother's milk is not available. Human milk has many advantages, such as decreasing the risk of necrotising enterocolitis that occurs frequently in preterm infants. Quality control according to evidence-based guidelines is extremely important for the operation of a human milk bank. (⌕ 94)

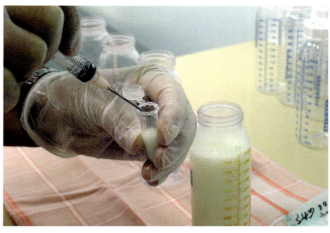

Fig. 120: Microbiological testing of human milk is essential when milk from donors is used [M307]

The potential stimulation of the immune system by means of an enteromammary path helps the preterm infants to produce type-specific antibodies. (⌕ 64) At the same time, by means of skin contact (kangaroo care), the infant transfers microbes to the mother. She in turn produces corresponding antibodies that reach the infant via the milk. The psychosocial effects of kangaroo care include improved bonding and positive effects on cognitive development. (⌕ 66–70) Kangaroo care can be an interactive measure to support self-regulation, that is reflected in the maturation of autonomic functions and in improved growth. (⌕ 71)

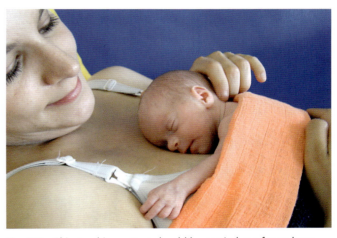

Fig. 121: Skin-to-skin contact should be carried out for as long and as frequently as possible [M307]

Postural stability, especially of the trunk, plays an important role in the oral feeding of a preterm or small for gestational age infant (SGA). The cheeks and oral-buccal fat pads, the latter of which are in sufficiently developed, provide the most stability during oral feeding. Therefore the preterm infant has a structural disadvantage. (⌕ 72) As a rule, the increasing capacity of the premature infant to be fed orally usually correlates with their growth and maturity. (⌕ 57)

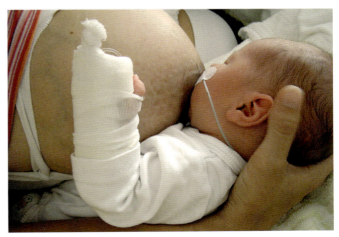

Fig. 122: The length of a breastfeed depends on the status of the child. Frequent, short feeds are less stressful [M307]

2.6 Infants with special needs

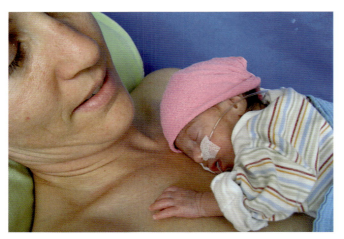

Fig. 123: Even if the infant nurses a little, it still obtains important experiences at the breast [M307]

It has been reported, that a preterm infant between approximately the 32nd and 35th week of gestation is capable of coordinating its sucking, swallowing and breathing abilities. All infants have an individual start in life, but small or delicate and sick infants that have been ventilated or have been very ill for a long time require longer periods until they are ready for complete oral feeds. (📖 57, 73)

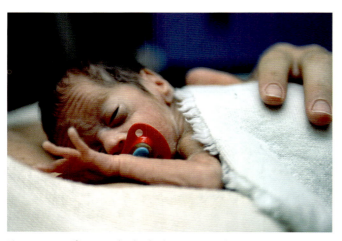

Fig. 124: Pacifiers can be looked upon as a therapeutic measure in preterm infants [M307]

Studies have shown that the development of non-nutritive (NNS) and nutritive (NS) sucking follows a developmental pattern. (📖 72) The NNS rhythm differs clearly from the NS rhythm, in which the infant must newly adapt itself to a bolus of fluid. A physiological sucking pattern, good lip seal, respiratory and oxygen stability, as well as a good skin colour are signs of an appropriate sucking behaviour. (📖 74–76)

Stability	Instability
Regular respiratory rate	Irregular respiratory rate
Good skin colour	Changes in the skin colour
Normal muscle tone	Hyper-/hypotony
State, for example, wakeful, attentive, but restful	Rapidly changing behavioural states
Hands active in the midline	Irregular movements
SaO_2 stability	SaO_2 fluctuations

Table 125: Behavioural signs and signals during oral feeding. Summarised according to Als, H. 1994 (📖 78); Sarimski, K. 2000 (📖 80)

Premature and sick infants frequently have difficulty regulating their behavioural states. The state of the infant is a combined occurrence of behaviours, which indicate its alertness. (📖 77–80) The reaction of the infant to its environment (e.g. stress, auditory stimulation and light) have an influence on feeding.

In order to progress with oral feeding, it is important that the infant be able to regulate their behaviour and state. A premature infant is often capable of good regulation at the start of a feed, though may have difficulties in maintaining this state up to the end of the feed. Parents and specialised staff must be attentive and respect the various signals given by the infant.

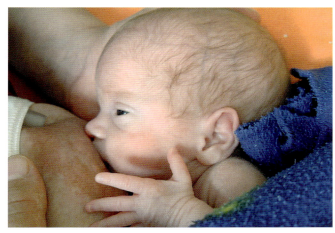

Fig. 126: The quantity of milk is (still) not important, the positive experience at the breast counts [M307]

International studies have confirmed the efficacy of various programmes, which acknowledge the importance of individualised developmental care for a positive outcome on infant development and on parent-child bonding, for example the Neonatal Individualised Developmental Care Assessment Program (NIDCAP). This programme for the care and treatment of premature infants takes into consideration, among other things, protection against noise and light as well as consideration for the sleep–wake states of the infant. (📖 77, 78)

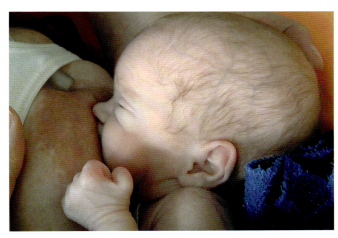

Fig. 127: Defensive state of the infant: A break may be required. Give me more time! [M307]

Premature infants often experience various forms of oral stimulation, for example, they are suctioned out, intubated, feeding tubes are placed and oral care measures are conducted. In the literature there are reports of a high percentage of former premature babies with feeding problems. (📖 81) Thus it is important that all oral experiences, whether at the breast, with the bottle or other alternative feeding methods, are positive for the infant. (📖 82)

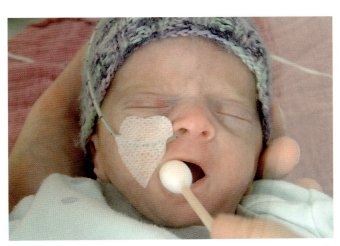

Fig. 128: During oral care, attention should also be paid to signals from the infant [M307]

2.6 Infants with special needs

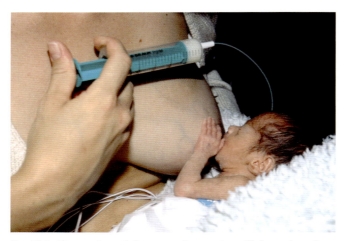

Fig. 129: The newborn infant experiences the milk from the tube feed and at the same time can suckle at the breast [E281]

The decision to start breastfeeding or oral feeding should be made on the basis of the individual state and health of the infant and should not necessarily be dependent on the gestational age or weight.

It is important for the infant to experience each new oral stimulus individually and at their own pace. This enables the infant to adapt more readily. (📖 58)

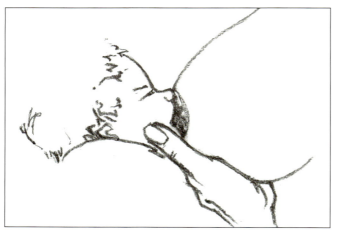

Fig. 130: Supporting the breast helps the infant to latch onto the breast [E281]

Most preterm or sick newborn infants require positioning that is individually adapted before they are able to feed. For example, it may be necessary for the mother to support the breast. By means of these measures, the infant can be supported in breathing and in the coordination of breathing and sucking patterns. With increasing maturity, the breastfeeding behaviour of the infant usually continues to improve and tube feeds become less frequent.

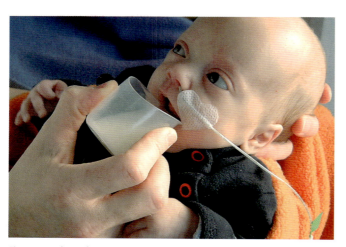

Fig. 131: The infant takes an active part. Postural stability is important [E281]

On many neonatal units, alternative feeding methods are used parallel to breastfeeding, such as cup, bottle or finger feeding. Therefore, it is necessary to pay particular attention to the physiological coordination of sucking, swallowing and breathing. Consideration should be given to the flow rate as well as to bolus control.

It has been reported that the use of a nipple shield when breastfeeding a premature infant increases milk transfer by about 75%. (👉 83) But, as with older infants, not every premature baby needs a nipple shield. Each situation must be individually assessed before a nipple shield is used. If milk does not flow spontaneously into the nipple shield before the infant latches on, the mother may have to express some milk into the shield.

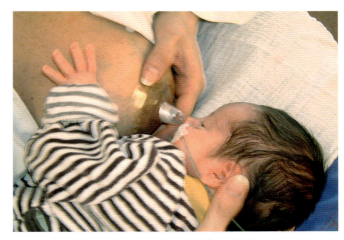

Fig. 132: Nipple shields can improve milk intake in premature infants [M307]

2.6.2 Respiratory problems

Preterm infants frequently have respiratory problems due to bronchopulmonary dysplasia or chronic lung disease. However, various respiratory problems can also occur in full term newborns and older infants. The focus of a child with tachypnoea and oxygen requirement is on their breathing. In order to support oxygen saturation and feeding, individual positioning, often with the infant elevated and the head, neck and trunk supported, is of central importance.

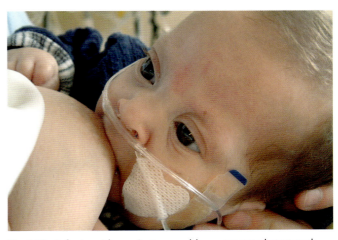

Fig. 133: Infants with respiratory problems cannot always suck efficiently and strongly [M307]

Older children often suffer from respiratory tract infections. This can also affect the breastfeeding dyad, because under these circumstances the infant is not always able to drink the usual quantity, which can result in a decrease in the mother's milk production. Frequent short breastfeeds may be necessary in order to help the child and to maintain milk production. Occasionally, it may also be necessary for milk to be expressed over a short period even in addition to or instead of breastfeeding.

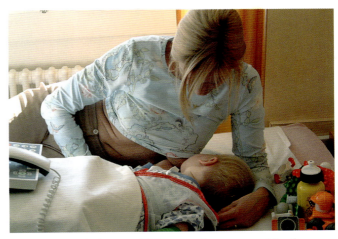

Fig. 134: Older babies or children usually recover quicker from illness when breastfed [M307]

2.6 Infants with special needs

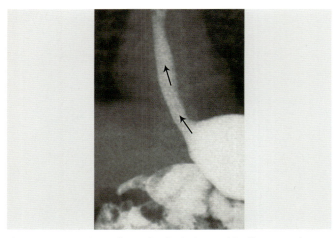

Fig. 135: A massive reflux episode during a videofluoroscopic swallowing study (VFSS). Reflux can result in oesophagitis and feeding difficulties [T348]

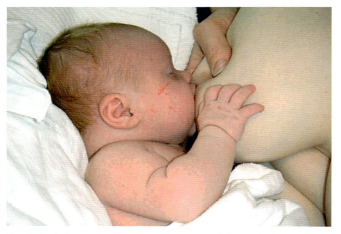

Fig. 136: Infants with Down syndrome profit from the breast being supported during breastfeeding [M308]

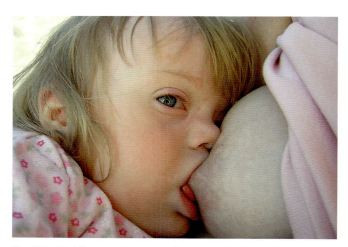

Fig. 137: Toddler with Down syndrome: optimal attachment promotes buccal development [O450]

2.6.3 Reflux

In a significant number of premature infants and occasionally in other newborn babies, gastro-oesophageal reflux (GOR) occurs, which can contribute to feeding difficulties. Some infants can be treated with medication, while, in others, symptoms such as hiccups, discomfort and oesophageal regurgitation disappear with increasing maturity.
It is advisable to pay particular attention to signals conveyed by the infant and to give structural support during feeds. This means to have the infant in an elevated position with the head, neck and back well supported. The infant's head end of the bed is often raised to an angle of 30°. (📖 72)

2.6.4 Down syndrome

With respect to both preterm infants and also full term infants with Down syndrome, some mothers are incorrectly told that their child cannot be breastfed. Because an infant with Down syndrome is usually hypotonic and oral motor development is weak, most mothers must initially express milk in order to achieve optimal milk production. If milk expression is required, dual expression with a full automic electric hospital grade pump is recommended, because it saves time and effort.

Breastfeeding stimulates the activation of muscle tone in the lips, mouth and tongue. The energy used should be kept as low as possible, because children with Down syndrome tend to have a slower rate of weight gain. If the mother has a large quantity of milk, she can skim the excess milk and give the fatty milk to the child, for example, on a spoon. In this way, the child receives additional energy (calories) for extra weight gain.

Special attention must be paid to positioning in infants with Down syndrome. During breastfeeding, it is advantageous for the head, neck and trunk to be well supported. The dancer hold for supporting the breast has been proven worthwhile. Until the infant has learned to drink efficiently at the breast and is putting on weight satisfactorily, alternative feeding methods may be required. Finger feeding is a common choice. As a rule, finger feeding enables tube feeding to be reduced or it can even be done away with completely.

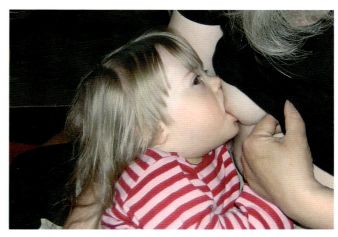

Fig. 138: Breastfeeding promotes a degree of 'normality' [O450]

2.6.5 Neurological impairment

Reasons for neurological impairment in infants include perinatal asphyxia, congenital neurological defects, for example due to a syndrome, or injuries at birth. The extent to which neurologically impaired infants are able to be breastfed is extremely variable. Some are able to drink well from the breast, some cannot drink at all, and some can only deal with small quantities of fluid from the breast or bottle. With neurologically impaired infants, throughout the feed attention must especially be given to an optimal, individually adapted feeding position, in order to avoid potential aspiration.

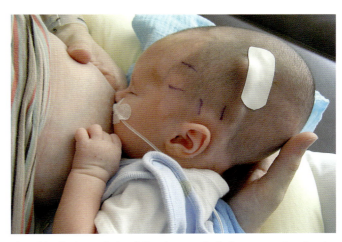

Fig. 139: Hydrocephalus following surgical placement of a shunt. The child and breast must be well supported [M307]

2.6.6 Cephalhaematoma (caput succedaneum)

During the birth process, small vessels between the cranial bones and the periosteum can tear. This can result in the development of a cephalhaematoma resulting in oedema of the soft tissues of the scalp. As a rule, the haematoma is resorbed within a few weeks and usually does not require treatment. Because the infant is sensitive to pressure and pain at the affected site, it is necessary to make sure that this area is protected during breastfeeding.

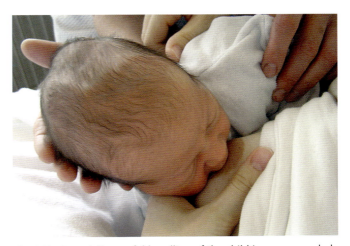

Fig. 140: Especially careful handling of the child is recommended in a case of cephalhaematoma [M307]

2.6 Infants with special needs

2.6.7 Failure to thrive

Infants that fail to thrive are usually indicating that something is 'not right'. Failure to thrive can occur in the neonatal period or later. Pathological or neuropathological disorders in infants can manifest as difficulties with breastfeeding or slow weight gain. In some cases the infants require (additional) feeding supplements. In addition, the mother requires sensitive support in order to maintain or increase her milk production.

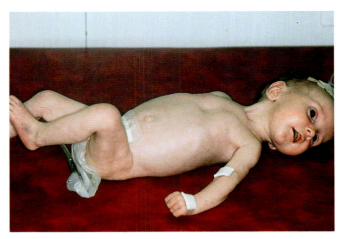

Fig. 141: 6-week-old infant, fully breastfed, with pseudo-hypoaldosteronism [O445]

2.6.8 Cleft lip, cleft of the upper alveolar ridge (gum) and palate

Cleft defects occur in in approximately one child out of 500–700 live births in Europe and most parts of the world. Part of embryonic development does not follow the normal pattern and results in a cleft defect. Clefts of the lips or the hard and/or soft palate can occur, both unilaterally and bilaterally. These clefts are associated with a syndrome only in rare cases. Most infants with cleft lip, alveolar ridge or palate are usually otherwise healthy and have no other defects. Male infants are affected more frequently than female infants.

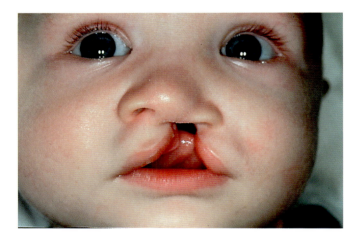

Fig. 142: Infant with complete unilateral cleft lip and palate. Breastfeeding was not possible [M307]

Infants with a cleft lip can usually be breastfed. According to their extent, cleft palates can cause substantially more problems with breastfeeding. Taking folic acid before and during pregnancy is recommended as prophylaxis against cleft defects.

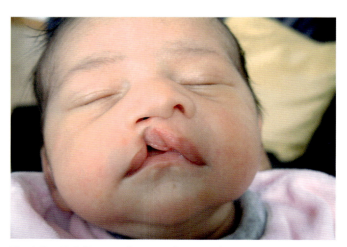

Fig. 143: Cleft lips usually cause fewer problems with breastfeeding [M307]

The use of a palatal obturator depends on the severity of a cleft in the hard/soft palate and respective hospital policies. These oral feeding obturators are made of soft or hard plastic and are usually custom fitted in the first week of life. An obturator separates the oral and nasal cavities and thus supports fluid/food intake during feeds. In addition, they prevent the tongue from continually lying in the cleft.

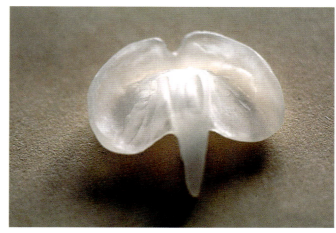

Fig. 144: Palatal obturator made of hard plastic. The fit must be checked regularly (pressure points snug fit!) [M307]

Regardless of the severity of the cleft, the infant should be nursed early while still in delivery room. These early experiences at the breast often influence the following breastfeeding success. The parents require sensitive and detailed advice on feeding. This should include the advantages of breastfeeding and human milk, for example, its immunological components, the fact that otitis media occurs only seldom, optimised development of the orofacial muscles, as well as the emotional aspects of breastfeeding. (84)

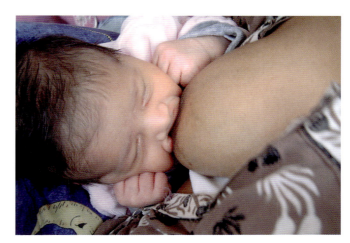

Fig. 145: Infant with unilateral cleft lip [M307]

In the case of a severe cleft defect, the mother should start to express her milk as soon as possible after the delivery. Initially, breastfeeding should not be seen as the focal point; the prime focus should be the development and maintenance of milk production. In all cases, regular experiences at the breast are valuable for the subsequent breastfeeding relationship. There are various alternative feeding methods to support breastfeeding, for example nipple shields, finger feeders and Haberman Feeders (Special Needs Feeder). (85)

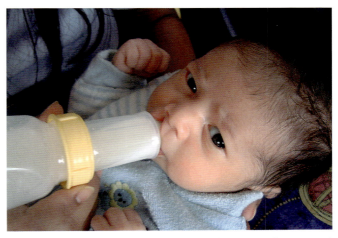

Fig. 146: Until the age of six weeks, bottle feeding with expressed breast milk was necessary (Haberman Feeder) [M307]

2.6 Infants with special needs

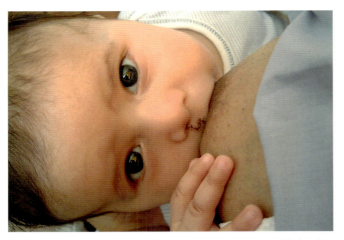

Fig. 147: 40 minutes after surgery for lip closure, the child drank 140 mL from the breast [M307]

Very different policies exist worldwide for the surgical correction of clefts. Cleft lips are mostly closed at the age of approximately 3–5 months, while surgical correction of cleft palates and upper alveolar ridge takes place at the age of 7–18 months. Mothers are usually very interested in obtaining precise information about the hospital stay, their involvement and the procedures, as well as how long before and after surgery they will be unable to breastfeed.

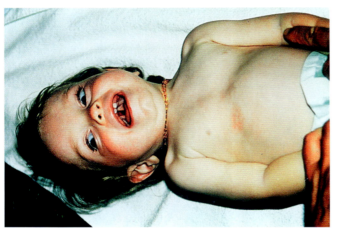

Fig. 148: Infant with a complete cleft of the hard and soft palate. Breastfeeding was not possible [M307]

Some babies with a cleft never manage to drink from the breast or bottle. There are cases where an infant has to be fed by tube with expressed breast milk for many months. Other children are fed using alternative methods, for example finger feeding, and then move directly to solid food (as in the case of the pictured child). The importance of professional and continuous support and instruction for the family during this often difficult phase of life should not be underestimated.

2.6.9 Pierre Robin sequence

Congenital Pierre Robin sequence manifests as retrognathia, which causes the tongue to be posteriorly positioned in the oral cavity, this can lead to obstruction of the pharngeal airway. In addition, a wide cleft occurs in the hard palate. The affected infants usually have massive problems with oral feeding and can only be breastfed in rare cases. In many patients, additional health problems occur.

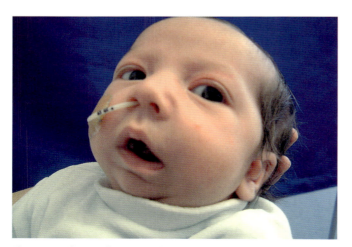

Fig. 149: Infant with Pierre Robin sequence and palatal obturator. Breastfeeding was not possible [M307]

2.6.10 Choanal atresia and stenosis

This is a congenital defect with a narrowing of the tissue membrane (stenosis) or a closure (atresia) of the nasal respiratory passages. The defect can occur unilaterally (more frequent) or bilaterally. Both forms can result in severe breathing problems and consequent feeding difficulties. Surgical correction is usually necessary, with the use of stents that remain implanted for several weeks until the respiratory passages remain patent.

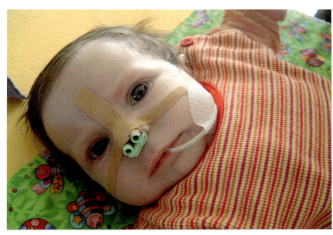

Fig. 150: Due to severe respiratory problems, breastfeeding was not possible. Feeding with expressed milk [M307]

The extent to which an affected infant is capable of oral feeding depends on the severity of the defect and can vary greatly. Some infants can be breastfed, but in addition require tube feeds in order to support their respiratory status. Some children learn to adapt their feeding tempo at the breast and to pause frequently and can be breastfed fully.

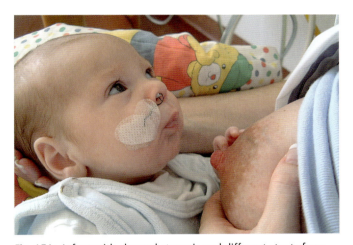

Fig. 151: Infant with choanal stenosis and different stents from Fig. 150 [M307]

It is very important to maintain the mother's milk supply in a sufficient quantity if the infant is not able to drink the necessary amount from the breast. A full automatic hospital grade electric dual pump is recommended in this case, because it saves time and energy. An individual pumping schedule adapted to the mother must be established.

In order to support the impaired respiration of the infant, it is very important to pay attention to suitable positioning during breastfeeding.

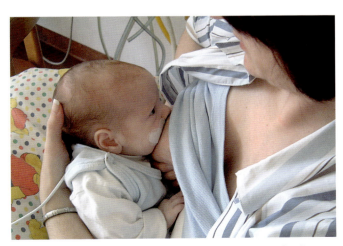

Fig. 152: Optimal support of the body facilitates breastfeeding. Small additional quantities were temporarily necessary by tube [M307]

2.6 Infants with special needs

2.6.11 Ankyloglossia

Ankyloglossia is a congenital oral abnormality caused by a shortened lingual frenulum. In many cases, the mobility of the tongue is impaired, which can cause problems with breastfeeding. These problems include grazed nipples, insufficient milk supply and a poorly thriving infant, which frequently results in weaning. Each mother–infant dyad must be assessed individually in order to decide on the necessity of frenectomy (clipping the frenulum).

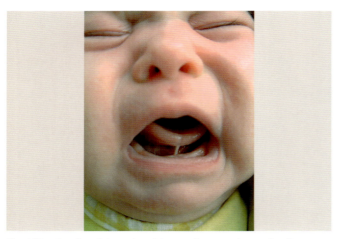

Fig. 153: Good weight gain with very frequent breastfeeding. Substantially longer periods were observed between feeding following frenectomy [M307]

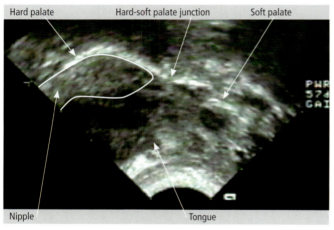

Fig. 154: The deformation of the nipple is visible by ultrasound (👂 86) [T349]

An Australian study (👂 86) showed changes in sucking movements in infants with ankyloglossia, with the aid of ultrasound. The objective of the study was to establish how frenectomy affects the sucking dynamics of infants. Before frenectomy, the child's tongue moved in a disorganised, piston-like motion with an accentuated upward curve in the posterior section.

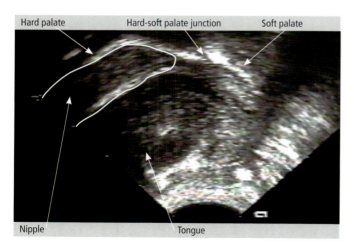

Fig. 155: After frenectomy, the deformation of the nipple is clearly smaller (👂 86) [T349]

After frenectomy, there is an obvious change in sucking dynamics and the course of movement is similar to that normally observed in a correct sucking pattern at the breast. In addition, the infants were able to empty the breast more efficiently and the mothers reported less pain. These ultrasound studies are an impressive demonstration of how a short lingual frenulum can contribute to breastfeeding problems.

2.6.12 Oral candidiasis

Candida albicans, the fungal pathogen causing thrush, is a commensal (normally harmless organism) and belongs to normal oral flora, and usually only causes problems when proliferation occurs in vulnerable infants. Infants with thrush often feed reluctantly from the breast. A detailed investigation usually shows white flecks on the tongue and the inside of the cheeks, which are not milk residue and cannot easily be wiped away. The severity of a *Candida* infection can vary markedly. In each case, it is extremely important for both the mother and the infant to be treated for a sufficiently long period.

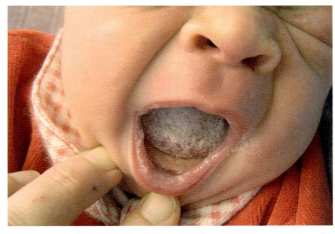

Fig. 156: Candidiasis following antibiotic treatment in a 4-day old neonate [M307]

2.6.13 Neonatal icterus (jaundice)

Neonatal jaundice is a symptom of elevated bilirubin. Bilirubin is the yellow bile pigment that is formed during the break down of red blood cells. Bilirubin is primarily excreted in the newborn's meconium. However, if the stool remains for longer periods in the colon, the bilirubin can be reabsorbed (☞ 1.7). Low bilirubin values are associated with early meconium excretion. (📖 87)

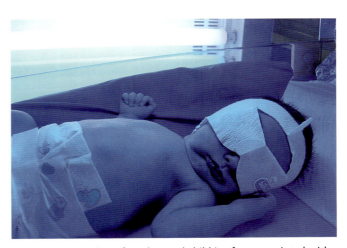

Fig. 157: Separation of mother and child is often associated with conventional phototherapy [M307]

Neonatal infants, especially premature ones, have an immature liver and often have higher bilirubin levels. There are various forms of jaundice and treatment must be individually determined in each case. (📖 88) There is no scientific evidence for the efficacy of administration of additional fluid in physiological neonatal jaundice, nor for a temporary pause in breastfeeding in cases of 'breast milk jaundice'. (📖 89)

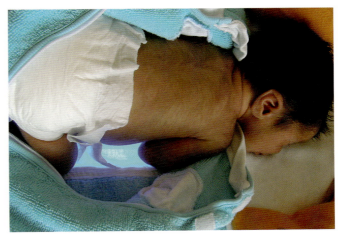

Fig. 158: An otherwise healthy neonate can remain with the mother, in its cot on a fibre optic blanket [M307]

2.6 Infants with special needs

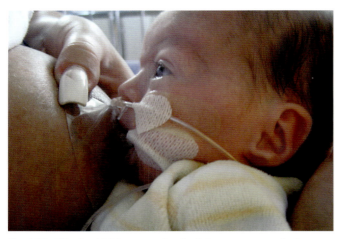

Fig. 159: Nipple shields can assist the infant to stay at the breast [M307]

2.6.14 Cardiac defects

As a rule, breastfeeding is less taxing for infants with a heart defect than drinking from the bottle, because the milk flow from the breast can be better regulated. Nevertheless, an individual assessment of each infant is essential. This also includes effective positioning and techniques that maintain good oxygen saturation and prevent aspiration. The infant can have problems staying at the breast and sucking can be weak and ineffective. The energy used should be kept as low as possible. (📖 90)

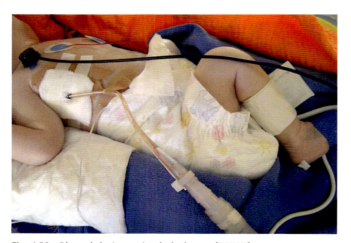

Fig. 160: Pleural drainage in chylothorax [M307]

2.6.15 Chylothorax

If the thoracic duct is injured, for example by a traumatic delivery or during surgery, chyle (milky, fatty lymph from the intestine) leaks into the pleural space and causes respiratory problems. Drainage and artificial ventilation is usually necessary. The affected infants require a fat-free diet with medium-chain triglycerides (special class of fatty acids) over a long period. It is useful for the mothers of these infants to express breast milk in the intervening period. Most of the time these babies transfer from the special formula to being fully breastfed without great problems.

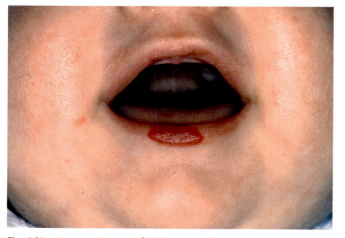

Fig. 161: Haemangiomas of the lips are often treated with laser therapy [T350]

2.6.16 Haemangioma

A haemangioma is a benign tumour consisting of a proliferation of blood vessels in the skin or mucosa. However, a haemangioma can also occur in the internal organs or eyes and cause greater problems there. Haemangiomas are mostly congenital and can disappear spontaneously. Haemangiomas of the mouth and lip region are of significance for breastfeeding. However, they only rarely impede breastfeeding.

3
Breastfeeding aids and alternative feeding methods

3.1 Aids for expressing human breast milk 60

3.2 Devices for nipples 67

3.3. Alternative feeding methods for the infant 70

3.4 Personal hygiene and clothing 76

3.1 Aids for expressing human breast milk

3.1.1 Breast pumps

It may be necessary to use a breast pump for various reasons. Given the diverse models of breast pumps available on the market, it is important to choose the one that is most suitable for each woman and her individual circumstances. Each woman should receive personal advice before using such a device.

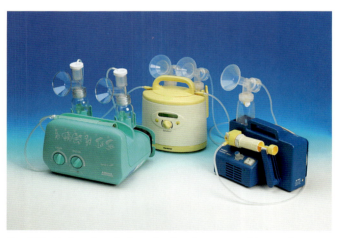

Fig. 162: Various hospital grade electric pumps with attachments [M307]

Electric pumps
Hospital grade electric pumps are recommended when milk expression is required over a long period, for example, when the mother and child are separated or when the child is unable to nurse directly from the breast. Fully automatic hospital grade electric pumps are also to be recommended for women with weak muscles or poor muscular coordination, because they make pumping less tiring.

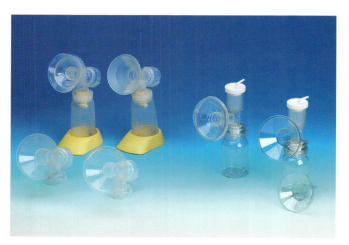

Fig. 163: The size and shape of flange is important for successful milk expression [M307]

In order to obtain an optimal result with the pump, it is important that the mother feels comfortable while expressing her milk. On no account should pumping cause pain, let alone injure the breast. (☞ 91) A flange that is too small or too large can not only decrease the success of milk expression, but can cause soreness of the nipple from rubbing. Advice on using a breast pump must include choosing the right sized flange to fit the woman; the nipple should be able to move back and forth easily during pumping but, at the same time, have a close fit to enable stimulation.

If the quantity of milk needs to be increased or maintained over a longer period of pumping, regular expressing is necessary. A pumping schedule adapted to the requirements of daily life can help in this. Particularly in the early days when a mother commences to pump, a fixed routine is often helpful. For example, breast massage, simultaneous expression for seven minutes, repeat massage, five minutes' expression, another massage and three minutes' expression.

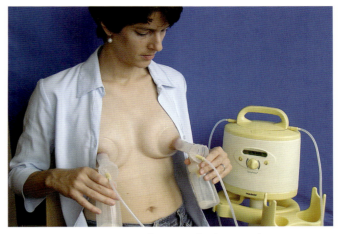

Fig. 164: Experience shows, for example, that simultaneous expression with massage intervals often stimulates milk ejection [M307]

Small electric pumps

Small electric pumps can be suitable for some women, especially for occasional use or for working mothers. Due to their relatively small size and low weight, they are easy to transport and can fit into a large handbag. Some but, unfortunately not all, models are also so quiet that they are not heard even when pumping in a discreet corner of an open-plan office. Battery-operated models have the advantage that they do not depend on proximity to a power point.

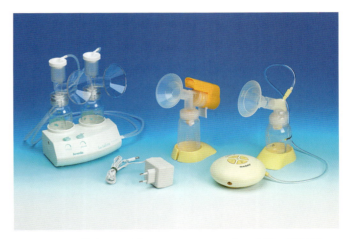

Fig. 165: Small electrical breast pumps permit mobility [M307]

Breastfeeding mothers in some countries are protected by legislation so that paid breaks for breastfeeding must be granted, there must be no work in lieu before or afterwards, nor may breaks be counted as part of the normal work breaks.

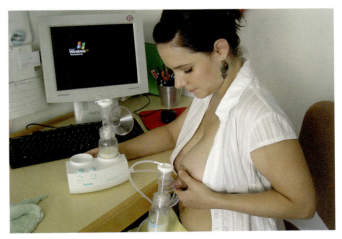

Fig. 166: Milk expression in the workplace [M307]

3.1 Aids for expressing human breast milk

Manual pumps

Manual pumps are usually cheap and are primarily suitable for occasional use. Their use requires a certain amount of strength and not every woman is capable of expressing large quantities of milk with a hand pump.

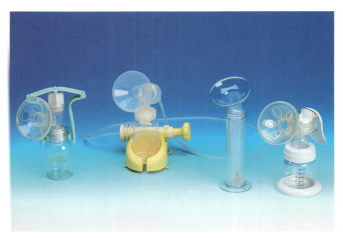

Fig. 167: There are many different manual pumps on the market, no one device is perfect for all mothers [M307]

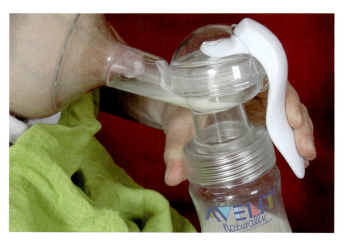

Fig. 168: Many working mothers are very satisfied with these manual pumps [M307]

One-handed models can be very effective with mothers who are proficient in their use. It is even possible to pump simultaneously with two pumps, or to pump on one side while an infant is being nursed on the other side. Further advantages of manual pumps are that they do not require any power supply and are small and quiet. These pumps are not suitable for women with poor hand coordination or problems such as carpal tunnel syndrome.

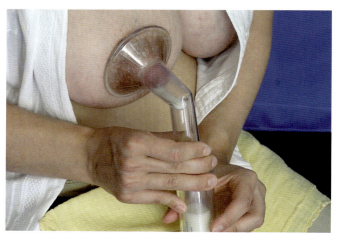

Fig. 169: An inexpensive model, which is however only recommended for occasional use [M307]

Cylinder pumps consist of an inner and an outer cylinder and work on the same principle as piston pumps. If the inner cylinder is pulled out, a negative pressure results, which causes the milk to be emptied from the breast. At the same time, the cylinder serves as a collecting vessel. These pump models are operated with two hands and usually the suction pressure cannot be regulated.

After each use, the pump set must be cleaned with detergent. First it is rinsed with cold water, then with hot water and finally with cold, clear water. In this way the milk fat is optimally removed. Once daily, the set is sterilised for five to ten minutes in boiling water or rinsed in a dishwasher at a minimum of 60 °C. Standard commercial steam disinfecting equipment is also suitable for sterilisation as well as suitable containers used for this purpose in a microwave oven.

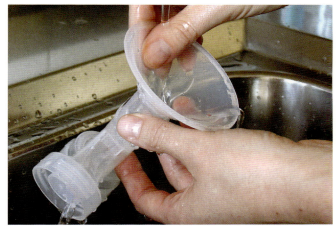

Fig. 170: Optimal hygiene is essential in order to avoid the growth of pathogens [M307]

When the pump set has been cleaned, it is shaken, left to dry on a clean dry surface and covered with a clean cloth. In this way, the growth of germs and bacteria are prevented. The cloths used for this should be used exclusively for this purpose. The pump set is not wiped due to the risk of bacterial contamination, but instead is air dried.

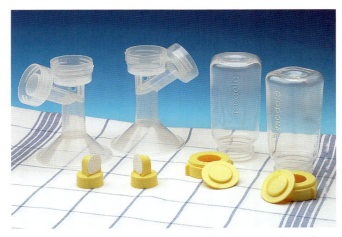

Fig. 171: Cotton tea towels are suitable for placing under and over the equipment [E281]

The rubber bulb pumps available for decades belong in a museum and not in the hand of a mother. Their disadvantages are so profound that they cannot be recommended. They are ineffective, difficult to clean and there is a high risk that the breast milk thus obtained will be contaminated. Moreover, there is no bottle in which to collect the milk. Since the negative pressure cannot be regulated, in the worst case, damage may be caused to the breast.

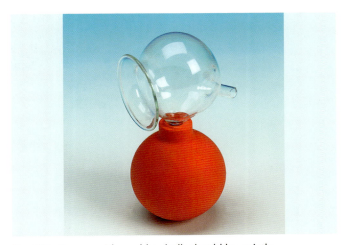

Fig. 172: Pumps with a rubber bulb should be strictly discouraged! [M307]

3.1 Aids for expressing human breast milk

3.1.2 Breast massage

There are women who, despite having an ample quantity of milk, find expressing extremely difficult. Manual expression can be a good alternative to pumping for these women. A further advantage of manual expression is that it does not need a power supply or costly equipment. As with pumping, the mother attempts during manual expression to imitate the rhythm of a sucking infant and to learn to stimulate her milk ejection reflex (☞ 1.2.3) when the baby is not at her breast.

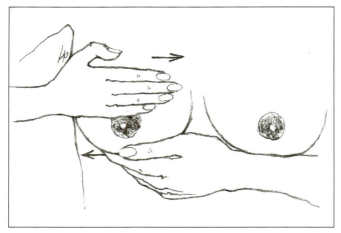

Fig. 173: The breast is taken between the hands and the glandular tissue is gently moved [E281]

It is essential that each technique for manual expression be gentle so as not to injure the sensitive breast tissue. Breast massage should precede the actual expression of the milk. During expression, the breast must never be pinched or pressed so hard that bruises appear. Likewise, the nipple or breast must not be pulled, since this can injure the tissue. Damage to the skin should be avoided, with the hands being placed firmly on the breast, with gentle tactile stimulation.

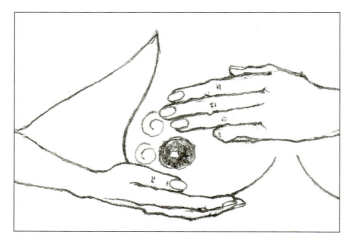

Fig. 174: The skin should not be rubbed during breast massage, rather gentle circular massage is used [E281]

Funnel for manual expression
There is evidence confirming that milk production is increased by breast massage and that the milk ejection reflex is stimulated more rapidly. (☞ 91) Some mothers prefer to have skin contact rather than to feel the plastic attachment of a pump. A collecting funnel is a most suitable and hygienic aid for collecting manually expressed milk with the least possible loss.

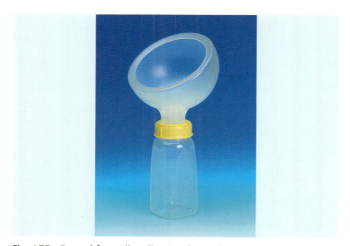

Fig. 175: Funnel for milk collection [M307]

A possibility for collection of milk while it is being expressed by hand is the Marmet Method®. This was developed by Chele Marmet, La Leche League leader and lactation consultant IBCLC. (📖 92) In this, one alternates between expressing the milk and massaging, stroking and moving the breast. The method can be used in order to express a small amount of milk, for example to relieve a completely full or engorged breast or to obtain a quantity of milk for a complete meal. The Marmet Method® can also be an alternative to expressing with a pump.

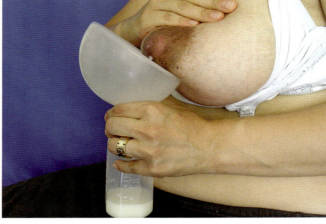

Fig. 176: A collecting funnel makes it easier to collect the milk that has been manually expressed [M307]

These small breast shields that may be worn in the bra serve only to catch milk leaking from the breast, but not in any way for collecting milk. For hygienic reasons, milk collected in this way should not be used for feeding and can, if required, be used as a bath additive. The use of breast shields in a bra that is too tight can lead to engorgement.

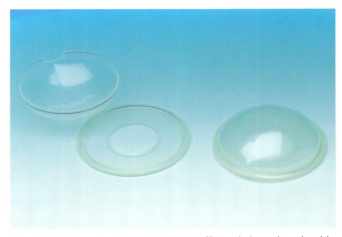

Fig. 177: While using breast shells, a sufficiently large bra should be worn [M307]

3.1.3 Equipment for transport and storage

Glass is the storage container of first choice for freezing breast milk, although it is subject to chipping and therefore used less frequently. It is the least porous material and offers the best protection for frozen milk. The second choice is clear, hard plastic (polycarbonate). Non-transparent hard plastic (polypropylene) is the third choice. In order to achieve the best possible protection, the storage container should be sealed with a firm, one-piece cover. (📖 93–95)

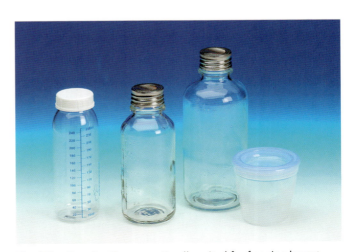

Fig. 178: Glass bottles are optimally suited for freezing breast milk [M307]

3.1 Aids for expressing human breast milk

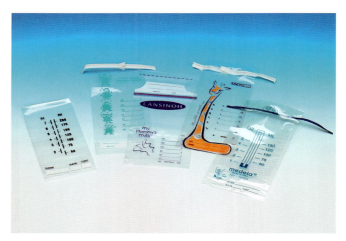

Fig. 179: Plastic bags are not always recommended [M307]

Milk storage bags require less space than rigid storage containers. In addition, they can be directly attached to the pump and shorten the time used to empty collected milk. The disadvantages of milk storage bags are: a higher risk of leakage than with rigid containers, the bag is less air-tight, there is a higher risk of the milk becoming contaminated, antibodies from the milk and milk fat can adhere to the plastic. Milk from storage bags is not suitable for premature or sick infants in hospital.

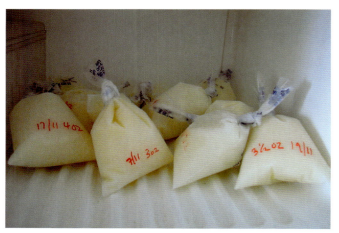

Fig. 180: Please, only for home use! Common household bags are not recommended [O442]

Freshly expressed milk should immediately be placed in the coldest section of the fridge. Do not place it in the fridge door! Cooled portions of breast milk collected over 24 hours may be pooled. The storage containers should be labelled with date and time and, if the infant is in hospital, also with the name of the child. Whenever possible, the milk should be used in the order in which it was expressed. It is advisable to freeze surplus quantities.

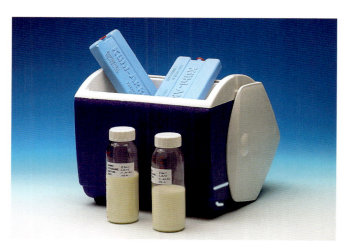

Fig. 181: Cool box with ice packs for transporting breast milk [E281]

Fresh, liquid milk is transported standing upright in a cool box with ice packs inserted in between. Bottles with frozen milk must be protected from breakage. Thawing should be avoided. For transport over longer periods, well-insulated containers with ice packs are suitable. The chain of refrigeration must not be broken during transport. As a general rule: one ice pack is necessary per full bottle of milk.

Milk that is pumped within one 24-h period can be pumped into the same container, if the previously pumped milk has been kept at a temperature between 0 °C and 4 °C. Transfer of the milk from one container into another should be avoided if at all possible, in order to keep pathogenic contamination to a minimum. Fresh milk can be added to frozen milk, if it is first cooled and if the quantity of fresh milk is smaller than that of the frozen milk.

The upper layer of the already frozen milk must not become thawed.

Table 182: Storage of a mother's milk for her own child. Other regulations sometimes apply to donated milk (📖 93–96)

Status of the milk	Room temperature	Fridge	Freezer
Fresh breast milk in a sealed container	• 24 h at 15 °C • 10 h at 19–22 °C • 4–6 h at 25 °C	• 3–5 days (at 4 °C or lower); • Store in the coldest part of the fridge (back wall)	• 2 weeks in a freezing compartment of a fridge • 3–4 months in a separate freezing compartment of a fridge with independent cooling • 6 months or longer in a separate freezer at a constant −19 °C
Breast milk thawed in the fridge, not yet warmed	• 4 h or less (until the next feed)	24 h	Do not refreeze
Breast milk thawed in a water bath	• Up to the end of the feed • Up to 4 h with continuous administration of breast milk by tube/pump	4 h	Do not refreeze
Warmed milk after the start of a feed	Up to the end of the feed	Discard	Discard

3.2 Devices for nipples

3.2.1 Breast shells (A) for inverted nipples

In principle, no nipple is unsuitable for breastfeeding, because the child does not nurse from the nipple but from the breast. A well attached child who latches onto as much as possible of the areola is important for breastfeeding success. Some healthy newborn babies are even capable of everting inverted nipples. Nevertheless, in the case of flat or inverted nipples, the use of a breast shell is often recommended. The success of using these devices prenatally is disputed. (📖 97)

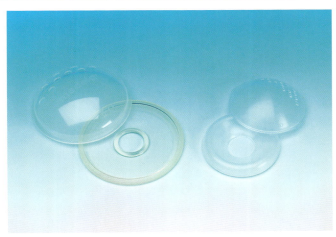

Fig. 183: Breast shells have a small opening in order to enable the nipples to evert through negative pressure [M307]

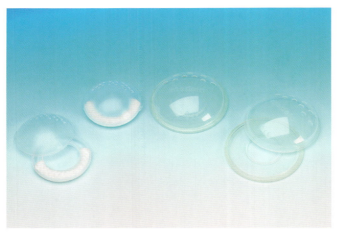

Fig. 184: The large opening of the breast shell prevents friction against the clothes [M307]

3.2.2 Breast shells (B) for protection

Breast shells can also be of assistance even when moist wound healing is recommended for the treatment of sore nipples (☞ 2.4.1). They prevent nursing pads or clothing from rubbing against or adhering to the already damaged nipples. In this way, pain is reduced and healing accelerated.

Caution: for hygienic reasons, milk that collects in the breast shells must, not be used for feeding! Drip milk is high in pathogens. (📖 94)

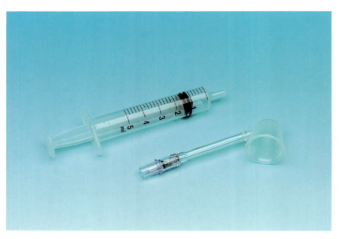

Fig. 185: Niplette for the correction of inverted nipples [M307]

3.2.3 Niplette

The use of a Niplette or similar new devices are usually designed for prenatal use, to evert the inverted nipple (☞ 2.2.2). The nipples are allegedly drawn out by negative pressure and, after continued use, remain everted. Many women find this suction device uncomfortable and its efficacy is not proven. Use is not recommended for mothers at risk of premature delivery. (📖 88)

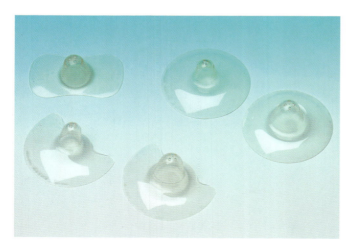

Fig. 186: Nipple shields with a cut-out section enable the infant to have contact with the skin and to smell the mother [M307]

3.2.4 Nipple shields

For a long time, nipple shields were absolutely frowned upon by breastfeeding counsellors. However, there are situations in which nipple shields may be useful. (📖 83) For example, perhaps to enable breastfeeding initially or to prevent a mother from weaning. The art is in recognising when it is useful to use nipple shields and when it is not, as well as providing professional support and guidance for the mother and infant. Nipple shields are not suitable as a quick solution for every breastfeeding problem.

If an infant does not succeed in nursing from a breast with a flat nipple, the mother requires counselling. As well as instruction in correct attachment and the handling and care of the nipple shields, the mother requires information on how to recognise whether milk transfer is occurring and whether her child is thriving. In some case, additional milk expression with a pump is necessary in order to stimulate sufficient milk production.

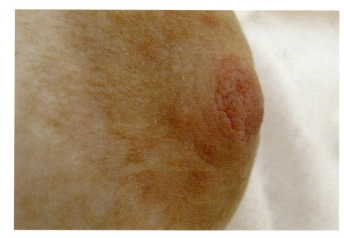

Fig. 187: In the case of flat nipples, the (temporary) use of nipple shields may be useful [M307]

Correct use of nipple shields

The nipple shield must be chosen so that it fits the baby's mouth and also the mother's nipple as best as possible. The nipple shield should guarantee sufficient intraoral stimulation for sucking.

If the nipple shield is too long, it can initiate the gag reflex in the infant and thus a defensive reaction. If it is too short, the nipple shield does not reach far enough into the mouth to stimulate the child to suck effectively. Correct attachment is also indispensable with the use of nipple shields.

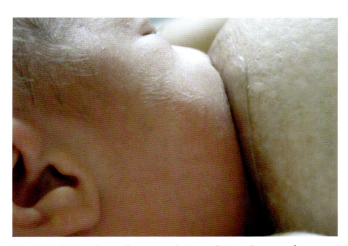

Fig. 188: Optimal attachment technique during the use of a nipple shield [M307]

Incorrect use of nipple shields

The infant must open its mouth wide, and take in not only the tip of the nipple shield but also part of the soft edge covering the areola. It is difficult to impossible for the infant to suck correctly and empty the breast efficiently if it latches onto an excessively long nipple shield and does not have part of the areola as well. Exceptions: sick infants or infants with heart defects, for whom contact with the breast is the primary function and the nutritional aspect less so.

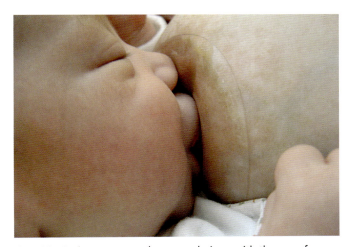

Fig. 189: An incorrect attachment technique with the use of a nipple shield can result in injuries to the nipples [M307]

3.2 Devices for nipples

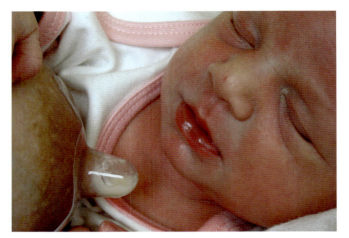

Fig. 190: A good sign after breastfeeding: milk in the nipple shield and a satisfied infant [M307]

There are publications stating that the use of nipple shields can have a negative effect on milk production. (👉 98) Many of these studies were conducted with the previously used nipple shields made of latex or rubber. (👉 99) Further well designed studies on the influence of nipple shields on milk transfer are absolutely essential, in order to reach definite conclusions regarding this problem.

3.3 Alternative feeding methods for the infant

In medical circles, the topic of nipple confusion is a matter of controversy, and is even considered not to exist by some. Nevertheless, both full term and premature infants can be hindered in successful breastfeeding by nipple confusion. (👉 87) During the first weeks, until the breastfeeding relationship is well established, it is advised to avoid artificial teats. Alternative feeding methods have advantages and disadvantages and are frequently not suitable for long-term use. In the ideal situation, all methods should promote breastfeeding and be practical for mother and child. Obviously, all resources should be used in such a way that the interaction between mother and child is maintained and promoted. All methods require instruction by a qualified person.

3.3.1 Cup feeding

The relatively less invasive method of cup feeding for administration of fluids is generally used above all in the early neonatal period, but sometimes also for a longer period. Occasionally, cup feeding is also used for preterm infants. It is important that the infant is held upright and plays an active part in drinking. The milk must never be 'poured' into the infant. Any cup with a rounded or flexible soft edge is suitable for cup feeding.

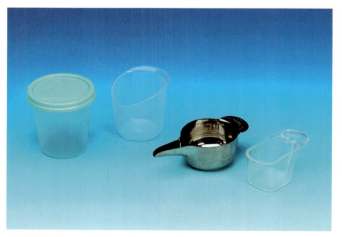

Fig. 191: Cup, Paladei, Foley cup: there are various vessels available for cup feeding [M307]

A cloth over the clothes of the mother or care giver protects against spilt milk. The infant should be awake and attentive. It is useful to swaddle the baby loosely, so that they cannot tip over the cup with their hands. Some infants drink without pausing, others prefer the cup to be tilted away between individual swallows. Several infants stick out their tongue while drinking, as if lapping the milk up. The mother should accept her baby's own style in cup feeding.

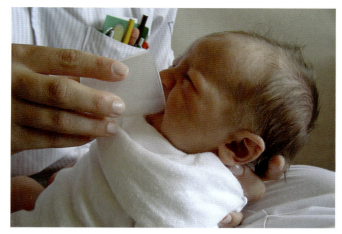

Fig. 192: During cup feeding, the infant determines the tempo [M307]

3.3.2 Soft feeder

A soft feeder consists of a bottle, a valve and a soft, spoon-like mouthpiece. The valve system incorporated into the mouthpiece enables the infant to control the flow of milk. The soft mouthpiece can also be suitable for infants with clefts (☞ 2.6.8) or other oral defects. The risk of breast milk being spilt during feeding is less than with cup feeding.

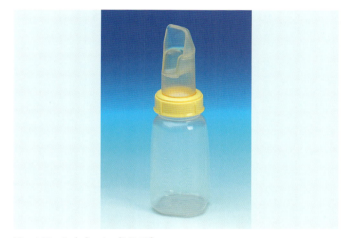

Fig. 193: Soft feeder [M307]

Many parents prefer the soft feeder over the usual cup, because it has a greater capacity and resembles a conventional baby bottle. Above all, when parents have previous experience with nipple confusion, there is a high motivation to use a soft feeder.

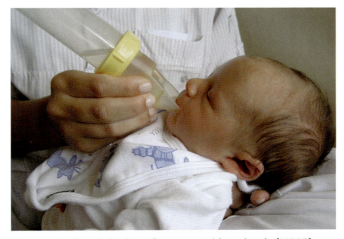

Fig. 194: At first sight the soft cup resembles a bottle [M307]

3.3 Alternative feeding methods for the infant

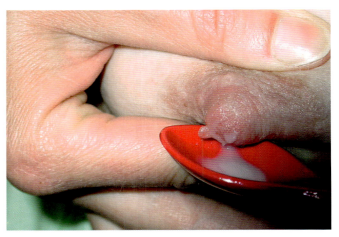

Fig. 195: Spoons are available in every household [O445]

3.3.3 Spoon

Feeding with a spoon is possible from birth and is primarily suited for the administration of small quantities of milk or medication. In principle, any small spoon is suitable, although soft plastic spoons are preferred. During spoon feeding, the infant determines the tempo. The spoon is placed at an angle to the infant's lips, so that the milk is licked off by the baby or trickles slowly into the mouth. Only when the infant has swallowed should more milk be offered.

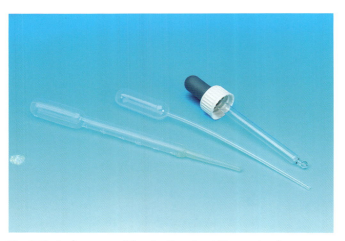

Fig. 196: As far as possible, pipettes should be made of an unbreakable material and hygienically acceptable [M307]

3.3.4 Pipette

With the help of a pipette, an infant can be fed both at the breast or directly. Soft plastic pipettes are preferable. The milk is either dropped onto the breast from above during breastfeeding, for example to stimulate the child to suck and swallow, or small quantities are dropped onto the lips of the infant. The disadvantage of a pipette, as with the spoon, cup and soft feeder, is that the child experiences no sucking satisfaction.

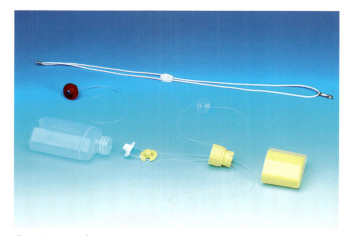

Fig. 197: Supplementary nursing system layed out with its individual components [M307]

3.3.5 Supplementary nursing system

Nursing supplementers enable feeding at the breast. It consists of a container for milk, ideally breast milk, or possibly another fluid, such as electrolyte solution, valve and holder, attachment, and two tubes (three different diameters) as well as a protective cover for transport. The container hangs from a cord around the mother's neck and the tubes are fastened with skin-friendly adhesive tape to each breast.

The supplementary nursing sytem set can be used short or long term. Its use lends itself to insufficient milk supply, infants with poor oral motor function, neurologically impaired infants, infants who are failing to thrive, during breastfeeding after breast surgery, when sufficient breast tissue is no longer present, and also for feeding of adopted babies. The use of a supplemental device requires good instruction and supervision by a qualified person.

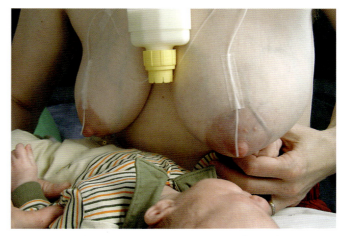

Fig. 198: Supplementary nursing system in use [M307]

It is important that the thin tube is positioned close to the breast and nipple, so that the milk can flow simultaneously out of the breast and out of the the supplementary nursing sytem. The infant associates drinking from the breast with a feeling of satiety. Although this device is quite technical, many mothers prefer it over the commonly used bottle, since they find it 'more natural'. In many cases, transition to complete breastfeeding is possible. (☞ 100)

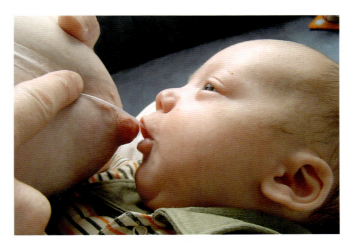

Fig. 199: Before attachment [M307]

The pictured infant was born at 32 weeks' gestation. Due to an embolism, the mother required intensive care. Although pumping was initiated early with a fully automatic, electronic hospital grade pump, milk production remained at a minimum: 40 mL in 24 hours at six weeks postpartum. Through the use of the supplementary nursing sytem, the breasts, and therefore milk production, were stimulated. The infant was discharged at 38 weeks' gestation and, after two weeks at home, was fully breastfed.

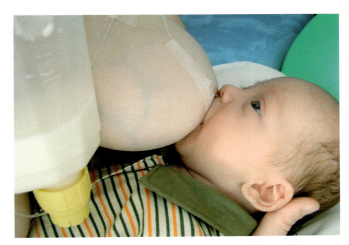

Fig. 200: A special moment (same woman as in Figures 14 and 65) [M307]

3.3 Alternative feeding methods for the infant

3.3.6 Finger feeding

With finger feeding, the infant receives a feed, or part thereof, while sucking on the finger of the mother (ideally) or care giver. For this purpose, a soft, narrow silicon attachment, or a feeding tube stuck to the finger is attached to a syringe filled with milk and introduced with the finger into the infant's mouth. Due to the use of finger feeding the orofacial muscle tone is strengthened, so it may be possible to reduce or even avoid gavage feeds after some time.

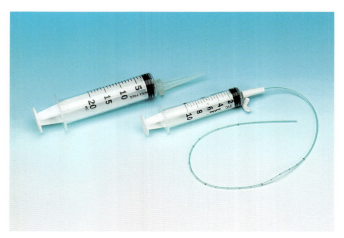

Fig. 201: left: finger feeding with silicon attachment; right with gavage tube [M307]

According to the age and gestation of the infant and fluid being administered, a smaller or larger feeding tube is used. The use of a feeding tube for finger feeding gives the mother greater freedom of movement compared with the silicon attachment. The tube results in less intra-oral stimulation than the attachment and may be more appropriate for an infant who has already had numerous oral experiences.

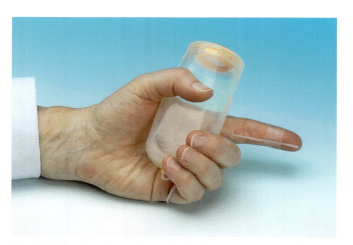

Fig. 202: The Hazelbaker Finger Feeder has an integrated silicon container (not available in Europe) [M307]

Finger feeding is not a routine alternative feeding method to replace the cup or bottle in the early neonatal period. The oral cavity of the infant is an exceptionally sensitive area and finger feeding should only be used when clear advantages for the infant and mother are present. Finger feeding should be conducted by the mother, if possible.

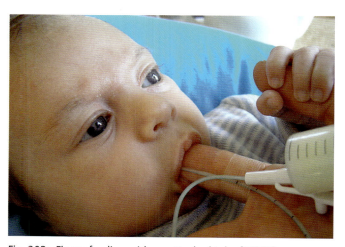

Fig. 203: Finger feeding with an attached tube [M307]

When finger feeding, it is important to support the infant well and pay attention to their body symmetry. An optimal interaction with the mother or care giver should be promoted. As with all other feeding methods, finger feeding should not be rushed. The child should determine the pace. Milk should only be given when the infant sucks and actively swallows.

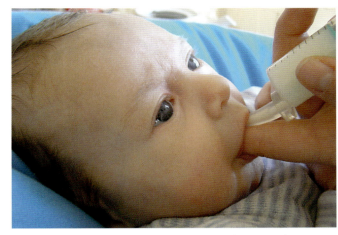

Fig. 204: Finger feeding with a syringe and silicon attachment [M307]

3.3.7 Haberman Feeder (Special Needs Feeder)

The Haberman Feeder has a special teat with a slit that was developed for infants with feeding problems, especially those with cleft defects. Since the flow rate can be well regulated, it is also used for premature infants. The milk flow rate is regulated through three graduations and a one way valve that simultaneously prevents the swallowing of air. The special size for premature infants is not available in Europe. Before a decision is made for the Haberman Feeder, it should be remembered that the teat is relatively hard, especially when it is still new.

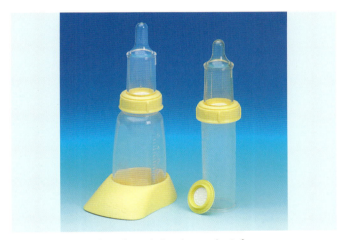

Fig. 205: Due to the relatively hard teat, the infant may use more energy; left standard teat, right teat for premature babies [M307]

When used correctly, the variable flow rate possible with the Haberman Feeder teat prevents the infant's mouth being flooded by a large quantity of milk. The correct placement of the valve plate is important, as is its immediate replacement when damaged. It is absolutely vital to pay attention to the correct handling of the Haberman Feeder.

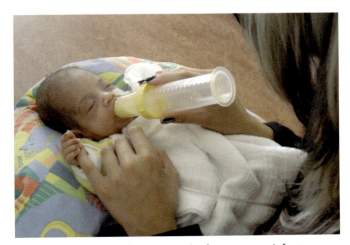

Fig. 206: Use of the Haberman Feeder for a preterm infant (standard size ☞ Fig. 146) [M307]

3.3 Alternative feeding methods for the infant

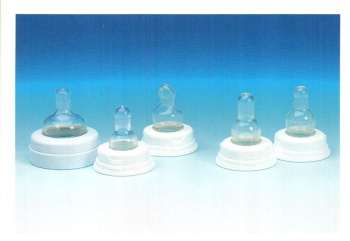

Fig. 207: There is no ideal bottle teat [M307]

3.3.8 Bottle feeding

So far, no teat has been developed that permits the same drinking process as from the breast! If bottle feeding is essential, a symmetrically shaped teat with a larger bulb-type base that is not too hard should be chosen. The hole in the teat should not be too large, so that the milk does not flow too rapidly. Even if bottle feeding, the side on which the infant is held should be alternated and attention paid to interaction in order to promote the infant's physical and cognitive development.

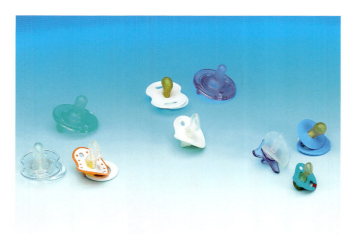

Fig 208: Pacifiers should be selectively used with a specific purpose [M307]

3.3.9 Pacifiers

As far as possible during the first weeks postpartum, pacifiers should be dispensed with, so that breastfeeding can become well established. If a dummy is used, it is better to use a soft and pliable product that has the smallest diameter possible in the region of the lips and gums, in order to have the smallest possible obstacle for mouth closure and development of the teeth. A flatish, rounded, symmetrical form is preferable. A bulbous shape (e.g. the so-called 'cherry form pacifiers') hinders correct tongue movement and encourages tongue thrust. (📕 101, 102)

3.4 Personal hygiene and clothing

3.4.1 Nursing pads

Nursing pads protect the mother's clothing from leaking milk. There are single-use pads and those that can be washed and reused. In each case it is important that the nursing pads are permeable to air and do not contain dyes or any toxic agents. Microfibre nursing pads are very absorbent and hardly wear out; pads from bourette silk have proven reliable for accelerating the healing processes with sore nipples. (📕 103)

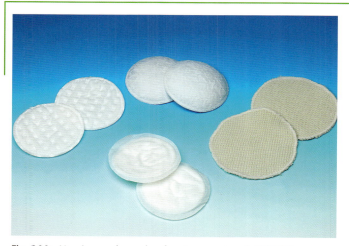

Fig. 209: Nursing pads made of various materials [M307]

3.4.2 Temperature packs

In order to enable breast milk to flow better, for example during expressing, it can be useful to warm the breast. In the case of breastfeeding problems such as engorgement (☞ 2.3.2) or mastitis (☞ 2.3.3), application of warm and cold packs can also be used. The ice and alcohol compresses that used to be recommended are no longer favoured and also the much recommended packet of frozen peas is not an optimal solution.

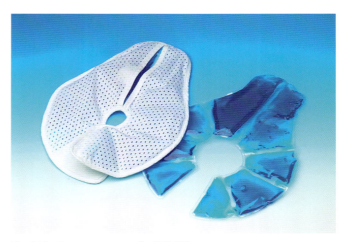

Fig. 210: Temperature packs [M307]

Reusable temperature packs can be used both to cool and to warm the breast, for example in cases of engorgement (☞ 2.3.2) or before expressing. They are specially formed to fit the breast well. In order to avoid skin irritation, temperature packs should not be placed directly on the skin, but always placed within a cover or wrapped in a cloth.

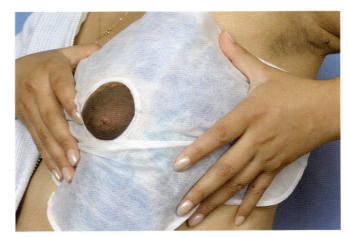

Fig. 211: The size of the temperature pack can be adjusted with a velcro fastener [M307]

3.4.3 Ointments

The cause of sore nipples (☞ 2.4.1) must always be determined and eliminated if possible. As long as the cause is not removed, creams and ointments can at best be considered to be cosmetic measures. If ointments are used to help wound healing, they should not be ones that have to be removed before breastfeeding. Thinly applied, highly purified lanolin is a tried and tested reliable remedy for sore nipples. (☞ 104)

Tubes or bottles with a small aperture should be chosen over pots due to possible pathogenic contamination from fingers.

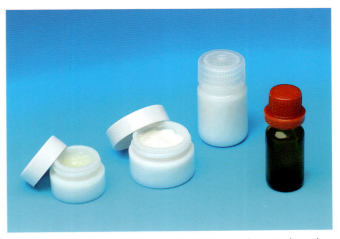

Fig. 212: Ointments and tinctures should be used sparingly and with a specific purpose [M307]

3.4 Personal hygiene and clothing

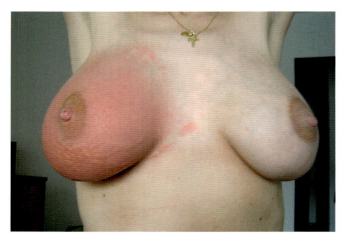

Fig. 213: Possible reaction to a poultice with salicylic acid, eucalyptus oil, peppermint oil and other substances [O445]

In order to avoid skin reactions on the breasts, it is advisable to first perform a skin tolerance test by applying a small amount of the ointment or tincture to a small area of the forearm. Allergic reactions on the breasts cause additional problems for breastfeeding.

3.4.4 Nursing bra

Many women feel more comfortable when wearing a nursing bra, especially in the first weeks postpartum. A well fitting bra is comfortable and supportive, while a poorly fitting bra can constrict the breast and may lead to engorgement, breast inflammation or sore nipples. Underwire bras are not recommended for lactating mothers because of possible pressure from the hard wire.

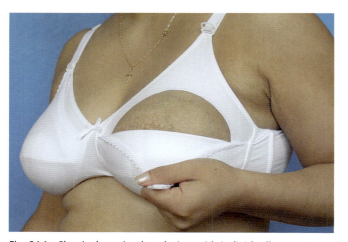

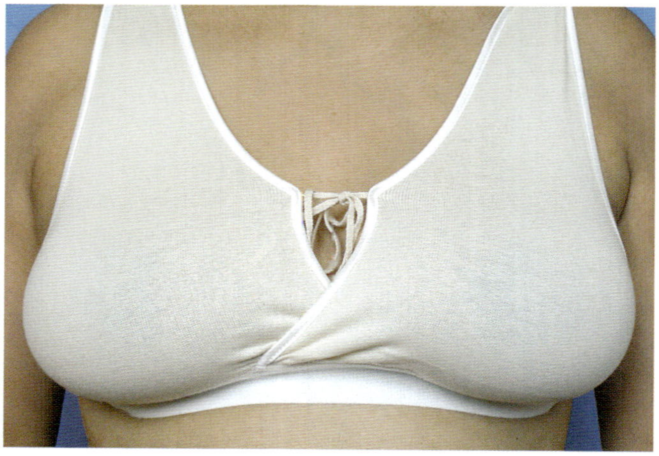

Fig. 214: Classical nursing bra design with individually opening flaps [M307]

Instead of a nursing bra, some women prefer a tank top or an ordinary elasticised bra that can easily be pulled upwards or downwards over the breasts. Natural fibres are preferable. A nursing bra is not a necessity.

Fig. 215: There are also nursing bras available made from natural fibres [M307]

Appendix

Glossary 80

References 83

Addresses 86

Websites 87

Index 88

Glossary

AAP: American Academy of Pediatrics

Accessory mammary tissue: ectopic mammary tissue that erupts in other places, usually along the milk line

AFS: Arbeitsgemeinschaft Freier Stillgruppen, an association of volunteer breastfeeding counsellors in Germany

Alternative feeding methods: alternatives to bottle feeding; ☞ finger feeding, cup feeding, supplementary nursing sytem, spoon, pipette

Alveoli: grape-like structures forming the secretory ends of glands; here: milk vesicles, in which the milk-producing cells are found

Amastia: absence of the breast

Areola: area of increased pigmentation around the nipple

Athelia: absence of the nipple

BDL: Berufsverband Deutscher Laktationsberater-Innen, professional association of IBCLC lactation consultants in Germany

BFHI: Baby-friendly Hospital Initiative

BSS: Berufsverband Schweizer Still- und LaktationsberaterInnen, professional association of IBCLC lactation consultants in Switzerland

C grip: method to support the breast while breastfeeding; the thumb rests over the breast and the remaining fingers cupped under the breast, each about 2–3 cm away from the nipple

Casein: coagulatory milk protein of large particle size

Cluster feeding: typical behaviour of a young infant, especially in the late afternoon and early evening; the child nurses for a short period, stops, perhaps even dozes off, begins to drink briefly again, etc.

Colostrum: the first milk already produced before the birth, with a high antibody content; supports the infant's immunity and promotes the excretion of meconium

Creamatocrit: measuremenat to determine the fat content and thus the energy content of milk

Cup feeding: alternative to bottle feeding, suitable for newborn infants

Dancer hold: named after Danner and Cerutti; a special manner in which to hold and support the breast during breastfeeding, used particularly with hypotonic or preterm infants or babies with cleft lip and palate

Donor milk: milk donated by a mother for an infant that is not her biological offspring

ELBW: extremely low birth weight; premature infant born before the end of the 28th week of gestation, weight less than 1000 g

Embryotox: information centre for embryotoxicology, information service for medical personnel regarding medication during pregnancy and lactation, Spandauer Damm 130, D-14050 Berlin, Tel.: 030/30308111, www.embryotox.de

Engorgement: breast inflamation usually caused by the blockage of one or more milk ducts

Enteral: concerning the intestines, located in the intestines

Exclusive breastfeeding: the infant receives only milk from its mother or a wet nurse, or expressed milk, and no other fluids (including water) or solid food, apart from vitamins, minerals, or medication in the form of syrup or drops if required

Finger feeding: alternative feeding method with a therapeutic effect, instruction by a qualified person is absolutely necessary!

Foremilk: milk at the commencement of the breastfeed (☞ hindmilk)

Frenectomy: cutting of the lingual frenulum

Frenulum: tissue attaching the tongue to the bottom of the mouth

Galactocele: milk cyst

Galactogogue: substance which stimulates milk production

Galactopoiesis: milk production

Galactorrhoea: involuntary and spontaneous flow of milk

Gestational age: age of the fetus or newborn from the date of conception

Gigantomastia: extreme enlargement of the female breast, also called macromastia

Growth spurt: phase with a clearly increased need for breastfeeding

Hand (manual) expression: collection of breast milk by means of various massage techniques

Hindmilk: milk towards the end of a breastfeed (cf foremilk); the fat content of breast milk rises during the course of breastfeeding, there is no threshold that permits differentiation of foremilk and hindmilk

Human milk donation: human milk obtained by pumping or expressing, which is used for a recipient that is not the mother's biological offspring.

Hyperlactation: excessive milk production

Hypermastia: ☞ polymastia

Hyperthelia ☞ polythelia

Hypophysis: pituitary gland

Hypothalamus: part of the midbrain

IBCLC consultant: International Board Certified Lactation Consultant; protected job title for members of the health profession who have passed the international IBLCE examination

IBLCE: International Board of Lactation Consultant Examiners; organisation that organises and carries out the examination for IBCLC breastfeeding and lactation consultants

Induced lactation: stimulation of milk production without a previous pregnancy, e.g. for an adopted child

Initial swelling of mammary glands: the so-called 'coming-in' of milk between the 2nd and 5th day postpartum (lactogenesis II)

Innocenti Declaration: joint statement by the WHO, UNICEF and other organisations for the protection, promotion and support of breastfeeding

International Code of Marketing of Breastmilk Substitutes: document regulating the marketing of and advertising strategies for breastmilk substitutes

Involution: return to normal size, here: process of reduction of the breast after lactation

Lactation: milk production

Lactoengineering: alteration of breast milk by technical or physical procedures

Lactogenesis: development of milk production in various stages: endogenous regulation of lactation in stages I and II, autocrine regulation in stage III

LBW: low birth weight, birth weight below 2500 g

Let-down reflex: ☞ milk ejection reflex

LLL: La Leche League; international association of volunteer, female breastfeeding counsellors

Lobulus: lobule; here: subunit of the breast parenchymal structure, consisting of 10 to 100 alveoli

Lobus: lobe; here: subunit of the breast parenchymal structure, consisting of 20 to 40 lobules

Mammogenesis: development of the breast

Mastalgia: painful breast

Mastitis: inflammation/infection of the mammary glands

Mature breast milk: breast milk following the completion of lactogenesis II

Meconium: the first stool of the newborn infant

Milk bank: institution in which donated human milk is collected, tested, processed, stored and further distributed

Milk duct: (sinus) lactiferous duct, serves to transport milk, not to store it

Milk ejection reflex: let-down reflex; triggered by the suckling of the child or through manual, visual or olfactory stimuli; release of oxytocin leads to contraction of the alveolar myoephithelial cells, thus forcing the milk in the direction of the nipple

Milk line: a line of epidermis extending ventrolaterally on each side of the body from the axilla to the groin, from which the milk glands develop; in the event of incomplete development of the milk line during the embryonal period, supernumerary nipples and ectopic glandular tissue may develop

Montgomery glands: sebaceous glands in the areola that secrete an antibacterial-like substance

Mother's own breast milk: milk from the mother for her own child

Nipple confusion: a feeding problem observed in practice during a changeover between the breast and an artificial nipple, not recognised scientifically

Non-nutritive sucking: sucking not for the purpose of nutrition, e.g. sucking for comfort

Oestrogen: steroid hormone produced in the ovaries, involved in the regulation of all female reproductive processes, including, among other things, breast growth

Oxytocin: a hormone produced in the hypothalamus and stored in the posterior lobe of the pituitary, which has an important role in triggering the milk ejection reflex, 'hormone of love'

Papilla mammae: nipple

Parenchyma: organ-specific tissue

Parenteral: bypassing the intestines

Partial breastfeeding: the infant receives an undefined quantity of breast milk as well as additional feeds and fluids of various types

Perinatal: period around birth from the 28th week of pregnancy to the 7th day of life

Peripartal: ☞ perinatal

Polymastia: supernumerary mammary gland(s)

Polythelia: supernumerary nipple(s)

Postpartum: pp, after the birth

Predominant breastfeeding: breast milk is the infant's main source of nourishment. However, the infant also receives water, or water-based drinks such as juice, oral rehydration solution (ORS), vitamins, minerals or medication in the form of syrups or drops, or ritual fluids (in limited quantities). Apart from juice, this definition does not permit any fluid serving for nutrition

Premature baby: an infant born before completion of the 37th week of gestation

Primipara: woman who has given birth to one child

Progesterone: luteal hormone affecting the development of alveoli in the breast; assumed to be jointly responsible for the initiation of lactation

Prolactin: hormone produced in the anterior lobe of the pituitary gland with a direct effect on the mammary glands and milk production 'natural sedative'

Pumping: collection of breast milk using an electric or manual breast pump, e.g. when mother and child are separated, when a child is unable to nurse from the breast due to illness or malformation, etc

Relactation: renewed milk production after weaning

Supplementary food: any solid food offered in addition to breast milk

Supplementary nursing system: alternative to bottle feeding, instruction by qualified personnel is absolutely necessary

Transitional milk: milk produced in the early postpartum period after colostrum and until the final transition to mature breast milk

UNICEF: United Nations Children's Fund

VELB: Verband Europäischer LaktationberaterInnen, association of European lactation consultants

VLBW: very low birth weight; delivery usually before the end of the 32nd week of gestation, weight less than 1500 g

VSLÖ: Verband der Still- und LaktationsberaterInnen Österreichs, professional association of IBCLC lactation consultants in Austria

VSLS: Verband der Still- und LaktationsberaterInnen Südtirols, professional association of IBCLC lactation consultants in South Tyrol

Weaning (primary): suppression of milk production immediately after birth, mainly by means of a prolactin inhibitor (not undisputed)

Weaning (secondary): termination of lactation at any given time; natural weaning is a slow process, in which breastfeeding is gradually replaced by solid food. WHO, UNICEF, AAP and national Committees on Breastfeeding recommend breastfeeding exclusively for at least six months

WHO: World Health Organization; supports breastfeeding worldwide together with other organisations, eg. UNICEF, BFHI, LLL

Witch's milk: secretion from the swollen breast of a newborn baby, caused by maternal hormones

References

1. Bannister, L. H. et al.: Gray's anatomy. 38th edn., New York: Churchill Livingstone 1995, p. 417–424.
2. Cooper, A. P.: Anatomy of the breast. London: Longman, Orme, Green, Browne and Longmans 1840.
3. Ramsay, D. T. et al.: Anatomy of the lactating human breast redefined with ultrasound imaging. Journal of Anatomy, (2005) 206, p. 525–534.
4. Neville, M. C.: Anatomy and physiology of lactation. Pediatric Clinics of North America, (2001) 48, p. 13–34.
5. Lawrence, R.; Lawrence, R.: Breastfeeding: a guide for the medical profession. 6th edn., Philadelpia: Mosby 2005, p. 68–72.
6. Riordan, J.: Breastfeeding and Human Lactation. 3rd edn., Boston: Jones and Bartlett 2005, p. 67–95.
7. World Health Organization: Global strategy for infant and young child feeding – the optimal duration of exclusive breastfeeding. Geneva 2001. Online. Available: www.who.int/gb/ebwha/pdf_files/WHA54/ea54id4.pdf; 27.11.2006.
8. Kalkwarf, H. J. et al.: The effect of calcium supplementation on bone density during lactation and after weaning. New England Journal of Medicine, 8 (1997) 337, p. 523–28.
9. Kalkwarf, H. J. et al.: Intestinal calcium absorption of women during lactation and after weaning. The American Journal of Clinical Nutrition, 4 (1996) 63, p. 526–531.
10. Kalkwarf, H. J. et al.: Bone mineral loss during lactation and recovery after weaning. Obstetrics and Gynecology, 1 (1995) 86, p. 26–32.
11. Collaborative Group on Hormonal Factors in Breast Cancer: Breast cancer and breastfeeding: collaborative reanalysis of individual data from 47 epidemiological studies in 30 countries, including 50302 women with breast cancer and 96973 women without the disease. The Lancet, (2002) 360, p. 187–195.
12. Prentice, A. et al.: Evidence for local feed-back control of human milk secretion. Biochemical Society Transactions, (1989) 17, p. 489–492.
13. Wrigh, A. et al.: Changing hospital practices to increase duration of breastfeeding. Pediatrics, (1996) 97, p. 669–675.
14. Yamauchi, Y.; Yamanouchi, I.: The relationship between rooming-in – not-rooming-in and breastfeeding variables. Acta Paediatrica Scandinavica, (1990) 79, p. 1017–1022.
15. WHO: Evidence for the ten steps to successful breastfeeding. Geneva: Revised WHO 1998.
16. Wolff, P. H.: The causes, controls, and organization of behavior in the neonate. Psychological Issues. International Universities Press, (1966) 5, p. 1–105.
17. Ramsay, D. T.: Anatomy of the lactating human breast redefined with ultrasound imaging. Journal of Anatomy, (2005) 206, p. 525–534.
18. Brazelton, T. B., Nugent, J. K. Neonatal behavioral assessment scale. 3rd edn. Clinics in developmental medicine, No. 137. London: MacKeith Press 1995.
19. Perinatal Nursing Education: Nursing modules – understanding the behaviour of term infants. 2003. Online. Available: www.marchofdimes.com.
20. Spielmann, H. Schaefer, C.: Arzneiverordnung in Schwangerschaft und Stillzeit. Munich: Elsevier 2006.
21. Kersting, M., Dulon, M.: Fakten zum stillen in Deutschland – Ergebnisse der SuSe-Studie. Monatsschrift Kinderheilkunde, (2002) 150, p. 1196–1201.
22. León-Cava, Natalia: Quantifying the benefits of breastfeeding: a summary of the evidence. Washington: Pan American Health Organization 2002.
23. AAP (American Academy of Pediatrics Section on Breastfeeding): Breastfeeding and the use of human milk. Pediatrics, 2 (2005) 115, p. 496–506.
24. Stuart-Macadam, P.; Dettwyler, K.: Breastfeeding: biocultural perspectives. New York: Aldine de Gruyter 1995, p. 129.
25. Moscone, S. R.; Moore, M. J. Breastfeeding during pregnancy. Journal of Human Lactation, 2 (1993) 9, p. 83–88.
26. American Academy of Family Physicians (AAFP): Position statement on breastfeeding 2002. Leawood: AAPF, 2002.
27. Human Milk Banking Association of North America (HMBANA): Guidelines milk bank – best practice for expressing, storing and handling human milk in hospitals, homes and child care settings, 2005. Online. Available: www.hmbana.org.
28. Roseman, B. D.: Sunkissed urine. Pediatrics, (1981) 67, p. 443, letter.
29. Lawrence, R.; Lawrence, R.: Breastfeeding: a guide for the medical profession. 6th edn., Philadelphia: Mosby 2005, p. 350.
30. Basler, R. S.; Lynch, P. J: Black galactorrhea as a consequence of minocycline and phenothiazine therapy. Archives of Dermatology, (1985) 121, p. 417.
31. Lawrence, R.; Lawrence, R.: Breastfeeding: a guide for the medical profession. 6th edn., Philadelphia: Mosby 2005, p. 105.
32. Riordan, J.: Breastfeeding and human lactation. 3rd edn., Philadelphia: Jones and Bartlett 2005, p. 98.
33. Neville, M. C.; Neifert M. R. (Eds.): Lactation: physiology, nutrition and breast-feeding New York: Plenum Press 1983.
34. Neville, M. C.; Morton, J.; Umemura, S.: Lactogenesis. The transition from pregnancy to lactation. Pediatric Clinics of North America, (2001) 48, p. 35–52.

35. Kent, J. et al.: Volume and frequency of breastfeedings and fat content of breast milk throughout the day. Pediatrics, (2006) 117, p. 387–395.
36. De Carvalho, M.; Klaus, M. H.; Merkatz, R. B.: Frequency of breastfeeding and serum bilirubin concentration. American Journal of Diseases of Children, (1982) 136, p. 737–738.
37. Yamauchi, Y.; Yamanouchi, I.: Breast-feeding frequency during the first 24 hours after birth in full-term neonates. Pediatrics, (1990) 86, p. 171–175.
38. ILCA: Clinical Guidelines for the Establishment of Exclusive Breastfeeding. 2005.
39. Radtke, M.; Kewitz, G.: Blut im Stuhl bei voll gestillten, reifen, gesunden Neugeborenen und Säuglingen bis 6 Monate. Laktation und Stillen, 3 (2005) 18, p. 90–91.
40. Daly, S. E.; Owens, R. A.; Hartmann, P. E.: The short-term synthesis and infant-regulated removal of milk in lactating women. Experimental Physiology, (1993) 78, p. 209–220.
41. Cregan, M. D.; Mitculas, L. R.; Hartmann, P. E.: Milk prolactin, feed volume and duration between feeds in women breastfeeding their full-term infants over a 24 hour period. Experimental Physiology, 2 (2002) 87, p. 207–214.
42. Frischknecht, K. J.: Die Bedeutung von interdisziplinärer Zusammenarbeit. Laktation und Stillen, 4 (2003) 16, p. 154–157.
43. Rees, T. D.; Aston, S. J.: The tuberous breast. Clinics in Plastic Surgery, (1976) 3, p. 339–347.
44. Ahlers, R. Menke, H.: Fehlbildungen der weiblichen Brust – Problemstellung und plastisch-chirurgische Therapieoptionen. Hessisches Ärzteblatt, (2004) 11, p. 647–649.
45. Grossl, N. A.: Supernumerary tissue: historical perspectives and clinical features. Southern Medical Journal, (2002) 93, p. 29–32.
46. Bakker, J. R. et al.: Breast cancer presenting in aberrant axillary breast tissue Community Oncology, (2005) 2, p. 117–122.
47. Both, D.: Stillen nach Brustoperationen. Laktation und Stillen, 3 (2002) 15, p. 88–90.
48. Cadwell, K. et al.: Maternal and infant assessment for breastfeeding and human lactation: A guide for the practitioner. 2nd edn., Sudbury MA Jones and Bartlett 2006, p. 84.
49. Abou-Dakn, M.; Wöckel, A.: Mastitis oder Milchstau – Teil 2. Deutsche Hebammenzeitschrift, (2005) 6, p. 57–59.
50. Giersiepen, K. et al.: Gesundheitsberichterstattung des Bundes – Heft 25 Brustkrebs. Berlin: Robert Koch-Institut 2005.
51. Collaborative Group on Hormonal Factors in Breast Cancer: Breast cancer and breastfeeding: collaborative reanalysis of individual data from 47 epidemiological studies in 30 countries, indcluding 50 302 women with breast cancer and 96 973 women without the disease. The Lancet, (2002) 360, p. 187–195.
52. Amir, L.: Eczema of the nipple and breast: a case report. Journal of Human Lactation, 9 (1993) 3, p. 173–75.
53. Amir, L.; Hoover, K.: Candidiasis and breastfeeding. Lactation consultant series two, unit 6. Schaumburg: La Leche League International 2002.
54. Lawlor-Smith, L.; Lawlor-Smith, C.: Vasospasm of the nipple – a manifestation of Raynaud's phenomenon: Case reports. British Medical Journal (1997) 314(7081), p. 644–645.
55. Mothers Milk Bank at Santa Clara Valley Medical Center: Donor FAQ, 2004. Online. Available: www.milkbanksj.org; 27.11.2006.
56. Modest, G. A.; Fangman, J. J.: Nipple piercing and hyperprolactinemia. New England Journal of Medicine, 20 (2002) 347, p. 1626–1627.
57. Frischknecht, K.: Entwicklungsbedingte Bereitschaft zum Trinken. Anatomische und physiologische Voraussetzungen. Kinderkrankenschwester, (2005) 10, p. 427–430.
58. Egli, F.; Frischknecht, K.: Geborgenheit Liebe und Muttermilch. Ein Ratgeber für Eltern von Frühgeborenen und kranken Neugeborenen, rund ums Stillen, Abpumpen und Muttermilch. Sarnen, Schweiz: Balance Kunstverlag 2002, 2004 and 2007. (available from: The Swiss Foundation for Breastfeeding: Schweizerische Stiftung zur Förderung des Stillens: stiftungstillen@bluewin.ch, www.allaiter.ch).
59. Schanler, R. J. et al.: Feeding strategies for premature infants: randomized trial of gastrointestinal priming and tube-feeding method. Pediatrics, (1999) 103, p. 434–439.
60. Furman, L.; Minich, N.; Hack, M.: Correlates of lactation in mothers of very low birth weight infants. Pediatrics, 4 (2002) 109, p. 57.
61. Cregan, M. D. et al.: Initiation of lactation in women after preterm delivery. Acta Obstetricia Gynecologica Scandinavica, (2002), p. 81.
62. Hill, P. D.; Aldag, J. C.; Chatterton, R. T.: Effects of pumping style on milk production in mothers of non-nursing preterm infants. Journal of Human Lactation, 3 (1999) 15, p. 209–216.
63. Hopkinson, J. M.; Schanler, R. J.; Garza, C.: Milk production by mothers of preterm infants. Pediatrics, 6 (1988) 81, p. 815–20.
64. Schanler, R. J.: The use of human milk for premature infants. Pediatric Clinics of North America, 1 (2001) 48, p. 207–219.
65. McGuire, W.; Henderson, G.; Fowlie, P.: Feeding the preterm infant. British Medical Journal (2004) 329, p. 1227–1230.

66. Bergman, N. J.: Randomised controlled trial of skin-to-skin contact from birth versus conventional incubator for physiological stabilization in 1200- to 2199-gram newborns. Acta Paediatrica, (2004) 93, p. 799–85.
67. Bergman, N. J.: The physiology of skin to contact part 1 and 2. Neonatal intensive care practices are changing. La Leche League International Breastfeeding Symposium Bilbao, Spain November 17–18 2005.
68. Charpak, N. et al.: Kangaroo mother care: 25 years after. Acta Paediatrica, (2005) 94, p. 514–522.
69. Department of Reproductive Health and Research, World health Organization: Kangaroo mother care: a practical guide. 1st edn., Geneva: WHO 2003.
70. Hedberg Nyvist, K.: How can kangaroo mother care and high technology be compatible? La Leche League International Breastfeeding Symposium Bilbao, Spain November 17–18 2005.
71. Dodd, V. L.: Implications for kangaroo care for growth and development in preterm infants. Journal of Obstetric, Gynaecologic and Neonatal Nursing, 34 (2005) p. 218–232.
72. Wolf, L. S.; Glass, R. P.: Feeding and swallowing disorders in infancy. Texas Therapy Skill Builders (1992), p. 297–313.
73. Als, H. et al.: Individualised behavioural and environmental care of VLBW preterm infant at high risk for bronchopulmonary dysplasia and intraventricular haemorrhage. Study 11: NICU outcome. Journal of the American Medical Association, (1994) 272, p. 853–858.
74. Palmer, M. M.; Vandenberg, K. A.: A closer look at neonatal sucking. Developmental Care. Neonatal Network Vol. 17 (1998) 2, p. 77–79.
75. Palmer, M. M.; Crawley, K.; Blanco, I.: Neonatal oral-motor assessment scale: a realibility study. Journal of Perinatology, X111 (1993) 1, p. 28–35.
76. Palmer, M. M.: NOMAS Certification Course Lucile Packard Children's Hospital. California: Stanford University 2003, p. 26-28.
77. Brazelton, T.: Neonatal behavioural assessment scale: Clinics in developmental medicine. Philadelphia: Lippencott 1973.
78. Als, H. et al.: Individualised developmental care for the very low birthweight preterm infant: medical and neurological effects. Journal of the American Medical Association, (1994) 272, p. 853–858.
79. Wilcox, M. J.: Premature infants and their families. Development interventions. San Diego: Singular Publishers 1995.
80. Sarimski, K.: Frühgeburt als Herausforderung. Psychologische Beratung als Bewältigungshilfe. 2000 Hogrefe-Verlag GmbH & Co. KG. D-37085 Göttingen Kapitel 2, p. 37–53; Kapitel 5, p. 117–142.
81. Papousek, M. et al.: Regulationsstörungen der frühen Kindheit. Frühe Risiken und Hilfen im Entwicklungskontext der Eltern-Kind-Beziehung. Bern: Hans Huber Verlag 2004.
82. Wilken, M.: Warum willst Du denn nicht Essen? Frühkindliche Fütterungsstörungen nach extremer Frühgeburtlichkeit. Ergotherapie und Rehabilitation, (2002) 3, p. 9–14.
83. Meier, P. et al.: Nipple shields for preterm infants: effect on milk transfer and duration of breastfeeding. Journal of Human Lactation, 16 (2000) 2, p. 106–113.
84. Herzog, C.: Mit Spalte geboren. Born with a cleft lip and palate. Video. 2002.
85. Herzog, C.; Honigmann, K.: Lasst und etwas Zeit – Wie Kinder mit einer Lippen- und Gaumenspalte gestillt werden können? Medela, 1999.
86. Ramsay, D. T. et al.: Ultrasound imaging of the effect of frenulotomy on breastfeeding infants with Ankyloglossia. 12th International Conference of the International Society for Research in Human Milk and Lactation (ISRHML). Cambridge, UK: Queens College September 10–14 2004.
87. Wong, D.: Whaley & Wong's nursing care of infants and children. 6th ed., St. Louis: Mosby 1999.
88. Biancuzzo, M.: Breastfeeding of the newborn: clinical strategies for nurses. 2nd edn., St. Louis: Mosby 2003, p. 247–252.
89. De Carvahlo, M.; Hall, M.; Harvey, D.: Effects of water supplementation on physiological jaundice in breastfed babies. Archives of Diseases in Children, (1981) 56, p. 568–569.
90. Cadwell, K.; Turner-Maffei, C.: Breastfeeding A – Z – terminology and telephone triage. Massachusetts: Jones and Bartlett 2006, p. 141–142.
91. Jones, E.; Dimmock, P. W.; Spencer, S. A.: A randomised controlled trail to compare methods of milk expression after preterm delivery. Archives of Disease in Childhood. Fetal and Neonatal Edition, (2001) 85, F91–F95.
92. Manual Expression of Breastmilk Marmet Technique www.lactationinstitute.org/MANUALEX.html; 27.11.2006.
93. Milk Banking Association of North America: Best practice for expressing, storing and handling human milk in hospitals, homes and child care settings 2005, p. 20, available from: Human Milk Banking Association of North America, Inc. HMBANA 1500 Sunday Drive, Suite 102 Raleigh, NC, 27607 www.hmbana.org.
94. Guidelines for the establishment and operation of human milk banks in the UK. 3rd edn. September 2003. United Kingdom Association for Milk Banking. The Milk Bank Queen Charlotte's and Chelsea Hospital. Du Cane Road London W12 OHS also available from: www.ukamb.org.
95. Australian Breastfeeding Association: Storage of breastmilk for infant use. 1999 (available from:

Australian Breastfeeding Association, 1818–1822 Malvern Road, East Malvern, VIC Australia; or: info@breastfeeding.asn.au).

96. Mohrbacher, N.; Stock, J.: The breastfeeding answer book. 3rd edn., Schaumburg: La Leche League International 2003.

97. The MAIN Trial Collaborative Group: Preparing for breast feeding: treatment of inverted and non-protractile nipples. British Medical Journal, (1992) 304, p. 1030–1032.

98. Auerbach, K.: The effect of nipple shields on maternal milk volume. Journal of Obstetric, Gynaecologic and Neonatal Nursing, (1990) 19, p. 419–427.

99. Lawrence, R.; Lawrence, R.: Breastfeeding: A guide for the medical profession. 6th edn., Philadelphia: Mosby 2005.

100. Guoth-Gumberger, M.: Stillen mit dem Brusternährungsset. Deutsche Hebammenzeitung ElternInfo (2006) 16.

101. Furtenbach, M.: Die Bedeutung des Saugmechanismus für die Entwicklung von Atmen, Saugen, Kauen, Schlucken und Sprechen. WirbelWind (2004) 2, p. 8–9.

102. Furtenbach, M.: Der Einfluss des Saugens an der Brust auf die orofaziale Entwicklung und das Sprechen. Innsbruck: Kongress Laktation und Stillen 1999.

103. Stadelmann, I.: Naturheilkundliches Konzept zur Behandlung der Windeldermatitis, Hebamme 2004; 17:236-238 (Naturopathic concept for treatment of nappy rash, German Midwifery Journal 2004)

104. Spangler, A.; Hildebrandt, E.: The effect of modified lanolin on nipple pain/damage during the first 10 days of breastfeeding. International Journal of Childbirth Education 8 (1993) 31, p. 15–19.

Addresses

Academy of Breastfeeding Medicine

191 Clarksville Rd
Princeton Junction, NJ 08550
USA
Tel: +1 609 799 6327
Fax: +1 609 799 7032
E-mail: ABM@bfmed.org
www.bfmed.org

Australian Breastfeeding Association (ABA) with Lactation Resource Centre

1818-1822 Malvern Road
East Malvern Vic 3145
PO Box 4000 Glen Iris Vic 3146
Australia
Tel: +61 03 9885 08 55
Fax: +61 03 9885 08 66
E-mail: lrc@nmaa.asn.au
www.breastfeeding.asn.au

Australian Lactation Consultants Association (ALCA)

PO Box 4248
Manuka ACT 2603
Australia
Tel: +61 02 6295 0384
Fax: +61 02 6295 0384
E-mail: info@alca.asn.au
www.alca.asn.au/index.html

Center for Breastfeeding Information (CBI)

CBI in La Leche League International
PO Box 4079
Schaumburg IL 60168-4079
USA
Tel: +1 847 519 7730
Fax: +1 847 519 0035
E-mail: CBI@llli.org
www.llli.org

IBLCE

International Board of Lactation Consultand Examiners
7245 Arlington Blvd, Suite 200
Falls Church, VA 22042-3217
USA
Tel: +1 703 560 7330
Fax: +1 703 560 7332
E-mail: iblce@iblce.org
www.iblce.org

ILCA

International Lactation Consultant Association
1500 Sunday Drive Suite 102
Raleigh, NC 27607
USA
Tel: +1 919 787 5181
Fax: +1 919 787 4916
E-mail: ilca@erols.com
www.ilca.org

La Leche League International

PO Box 4079
Schaumburg IL, 60168-4079
USA
Tel: +1(847)519 7730
Fax: +1(847)519 0035
www.llli.org

Network of Australian Lactation Colleges

http://lactation.org.au/index.html

New Zealand Lactation Consultants Association (NZLCA)

PO Box 29-279, Christchurch
New Zealand
E-mail secretary@nzlca.org.nz
www.nzlca.org.nz/contact.html

World Alliance for Breastfeeding Advocacy (WABA)

Sekretariat
PO Box 1200
10850 Penang
Malaysia
Tel: +60 4 658 4816
Fax: +60 4 657 2655
E-mail: waba@streamyx.com
www.waba.org.my

World Health Organization (WHO)

Avenue Appia 20
CH-1211 Geneva 27
Switzerland
Tel: +41 (0) 22 791 2111
Fax: + 41 (0) 22 791 3111
E-mail: info@who.int
www.who.int

UNICEF

3 United Nations Plaza
New York, NY 10017
USA
Tel: +1 212 326 7000
Fax: +1 212 887 7465
E-mail: netmaster@unicef.org
www.unicef.org

Websites

Organisations and associations

- American Academy of Pediatrics (AAP): www.aap.org
- Australian Breastfeeding Association (ABA): www.breastfeeding.asn.au/
- Baby Friendly Initiative: www.babyfriendly.org.uk/
- Baby Milk Action: www.babymilkaction.org/
- Breastfeeding and the Use of Human Milch (RE9729): www.aap.org/policy/re9729.html
- Feeding Young Children (Recommendation of the WHO): http://www.who.int/child-adolescent-health/NUTRITION/infant.htm
- International Baby Food Network (IBFAN): www.ibfn.org
- International Board of Lactation Consultant Examiners (IBLCE): www.iblce.org
- International Lactation Consultant Association (ILCA): www.ilca.org
- La Leche League International (LLLI): www.llli.org
- UNICEF Facts for Life: www.unicef.org/ffl/
- UNICEF: www.unicef.org
- World Alliance for Breastfeeding Action (WABA): waba.org.my
- World Health Organization (WHO): www.who.int

Data bank

- PubMed-Medline www.ncbi.nlm.nih.gov/entrez/query.fcgi?db=PubMed

Mailing lists

- Lactnet: http://peach.ease.lsoft.com/scripts/wa.exe?SUBED1=lactnet&A=1

Sources of information and education

- Academy of Breastfeeding Medicine: www.bfmed.org
- Association for Infant Mental Health: www.aaimhi.org/
- Australian Government Dept of Health and Ageing: www.health.gov.au/
- Baby Friendly Education Program: www.babyfriendly.sa.gov.au/
- Breastfeeding Resource: www.BORSTVOEDING.com
- Breastfeeding.com - Resource for Breastfeeding Information and Support: www.breastfeeding.com
- Bright Future Lactation Resource Centre: www.bflrc.com/
- Cliparts for download: www.promom.org/gallery/index.php
- Drugs and Lactation Database: http://toxnet.nlm.nih.gov/cgi-bin/sis/htmlgen?LACT
- Food Standard Australia New Zealand: www.foodstandards.gov.au/
- http://linkagesproject.org/
- Human Milk Banking Association of North America: www.hmbana.org/index.php?mode=home
- James McKenna's website about sleep and co-sleeping: www.nd.edu/~jmckenn1/lab/
- Lactation Resources: www.pabreastfeeding.org/pabcres.html
- National Institute for Health and Clinical Excellence: www.nice.org.uk/
- ProMoM: www.promom.org
- The International Society for Research in Human Milk and Lactation: www.isrhml.org.umu.se/
- www.lactivist.com/

Journals

- Breastfeeding Review: www.breastfeeding.asn.au/lrc/bfreview.html
- British Medical Journal: www.bmj.com
- Dietary Guidelines for All Australians www.nhmrc.gov.au/publications/synopses/dietsyn.htm
- International Breastfeeding Journal: www.internationalbreastfeedingjournal.com/
- Journal of Human Lactation: www.sagepub.com/journal.aspx?pid=250
- Pediatric Research: www.pedresearch.com
- Pediatrics: www.pediatrics.org
- The Lancet: www.thelancet.com

Index

A

Abscess 35
Allergic reaction 39, 78
Amazon syndrome 27
Anatomy of the breast 2
Ankyloglossia 56
Augmentation surgery 29

B

Behaviour, of the infant 13
Bottle feeding 76
Bowel movements of the infant 21
Breast
    Abscess 35
    Anatomy 2
    Asymmetrical 26
    Augmentation surgery 29
    Before birth 4
    Cancer 36
    Development, during puberty 3
    During pregnancy 3
    Enlargement (augmentation) 29
    Massage 64
    Pathological deviation 34
    Reduction surgery 29
    Shape, atypical 26
    Tubular 26
Breast milk
    Appearance 19
    Blood in 20
    Deep freezing 65
    Fat content 20
    Mature 20
    Storing 65
    Transitional 20
Breast pump 60
    Cleaning 63
Breastfeed
    Ending of a
    Formula
    Milk funnel for manual
     expression
    Blood in
Breastfeeding
    After breast surgery 28
    After caesarean 16
    Positions 14
    Relationship 4
    Toddler 18
Breastmilk stool 21
Breastpads 76
Breathing difficulties 49
Brick dust sediment 23

C

Candidiasis 38
Cephalhaematoma 51
Choanal atresia 55
Choanal stenosis 55
Chylothorax 58
Cleft lip 52
Cleft palate 52
Clothing 76
Cluster feeding 4
Colostrum 19
Cradle position 14
Creamatocrit 44
Cross-cradle hold 18
Cup feeding 70

D

Devices 59
    For the infant 70
Down syndrome 55
Dummy 46, 76

E

Engorgement 4, 34
Expressing by hand 64

F

Failure to thrive 52
Feeding cues 10
Feeding session 9
    Ending of a 11
Feeding tube 74
Finger feeding 74
Football position 15
Frenulotomy 56
Frenulum 56
    Tongue tie 56

G

Galactopoiesis 20
Glandular tissue 26

H

Haberman Feeder 75
Haemangioma 58
Hand expression funnel 64
Heart defect 58
Herpes 39
Human placental lactogen 7
Hydrocephalus 51

I

Ikterus 51
Infection 39
Initial engorgement 4
Inverted nipples 31

L

Lactiferous duct 2
Lactiferous sinus 2
Lactogenesis I 3, 19
Lactogenesis II 7, 20
Lactogenesis III 8
Latch-on/attachment
    Correct 11
    First time 7
    Incorrect 11
Leaning over position 16
Let-down-reflex 12

M

Marmet Method® 65
Mastitis 35
Meconium 21
Menopause 6
Milk bags 66
Milk bleb/blister 40
Milk collecting funnel 64
Milk ducts 2
Milk ejection reflex 12
Multiple infants 17

N

Neonatal jaundice 19, 57
Neurological impairment 51
Niplette 68
Nipple
    Accessory 27
    Cancer 36
    Confusion 70
    Cracked 37
    Devices 67
    Double 33
    Flat 30
    Former 67
    Inverted 31
    Large 33
    Painful 37
    Pore 2
    Shape 30
    Shells 68
    Shields 49, 68
    Small 33
    Sore 37
    Split 33
    Wounded 37
Nursing bra 78
Nursing supplementer 72

O

Obturator 53
Ointments 72
Oral thrush 57

P

Pacifier 76
Paget's disease of the nipple 36
Parallel position 17
Personal hygiene 76
Physiology of the breast 2
Piercing 41
Pierre Robin syndrome 54
Pipette 72
Plugged ducts 34
Poland's syndrome 27
Polymastia 27
Polythelia 28
Premature baby 42
    Behaviour 46
    Oral care 47
    Pacifier 46, 76
    Sucking pattern 46
Prolactin-inhibiting factor 7
Pseudohypoaldosteronism 52
Psoriasis 38
Pumping schedule 61

R

Raynaud's phenomenon 40
Reaction, oral 10
Reduction 29
Reflexes, oral 10
Reflux 50
Respiratoral problems 49
Rhagades 37
Rooming-in 8
Rooting reflex 10

S

Side-lying position 15
Soft feeder 71
Spoon feeding 72
Stool
    Blood in 23
    Cow's milk fed 22
Storing of breastmilk
    Devices for 65
Straddle position 15

T

Tandem breast feeding 19
Tattoo 41
Temperature packs 77
Thrush 38
Transitional milk 20
Transitional stool 21
Transport devices 65
Twins 17

U

Urination
    Of the infant 23

V

Vasospasm 37, 40
V-position/double cradle hold 18

W

Weaning 5

Y

Yeast infection 38